John Josselyn, Edward Tuckerman

New-England's Rarities Discovered in Birds, Beasts, Fishes, Serpents,

and Plants

of that Country

John Josselyn, Edward Tuckerman

New-England's Rarities Discovered in Birds, Beasts, Fishes, Serpents, and Plants
of that Country

ISBN/EAN: 9783337308827

Printed in Europe, USA, Canada, Australia, Japan

Cover: Foto ©Andreas Hilbeck / pixelio.de

More available books at **www.hansebooks.com**

NEW-ENGLAND'S

RARITIES

DISCOVERED IN BIRDS, BEASTS, FISHES, SERPENTS, AND PLANTS OF THAT COUNTRY.

By *JOHN JOSSELYN*, Gent.

With an Introduction and Notes,

By *EDWARD TUCKERMAN, M.A.*

Boston:
WILLIAM VEAZIE.
MDCCCLXV.

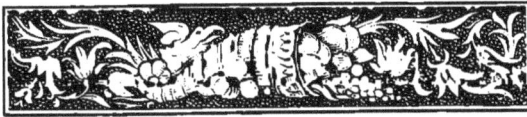

Publisher's Advertisement.

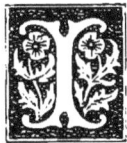

I N the reproduction of this quaint and curious treatise, which is one of the earliest, on the *Natural History of New England*, it has been the intention of the Publisher to enhance its value as a literary curiosity, by making it as nearly as possible an exact Fac-simile of the original edition, in accordance with the projected plan of a series of reprints, in which the present work is comprised.

In the furtherance of this intention, the precise orthography, punctuation, and also the arrangement, — with the exception of the commencement and termination of pages, — have been preserved.

The valuable Introduction and Notes of Prof. TUCK-ERMAN, incorporated in this edition, have been previously issued in vol. iv. of "The Transactions of the American Antiquarian Society," which contains a reprint of "The Rarities" in a more modern style. The notes have, however, undergone a thorough revision by the author; and some few additions have been made by him, during the progress of the present edition through the press.

Some additional matter concerning the Genealogy of the Josselyn Family may be found contained in the Preface of the "Two Voyages to New England in 1638 and 1663, by John Josselyn," published in uniform style with the present work.

BOSTON, MAY 15, 1865.

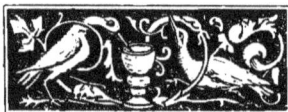

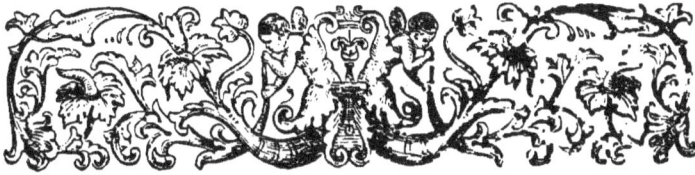

INTRODUCTION.

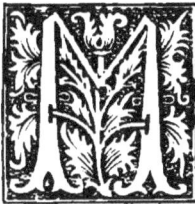

R. JOHN JOSSELYN, the writer of this book, was only brother, as he fays, to Henry Joffelyn, Efq., many years of Black Point in Scarborough, Me.; and both were fons to Sir Thomas Joffelyn, Knt., of Kent, whofe name is at the head of the new charter obtained by Sir Ferdinando Gorges for his Province in 1639, but who did not come to this country. Mr. Henry Joffelyn was at Pifcataqua, in the intereft of Capt. John Mafon, at leaft as early as 1634; but, in 1636, he is one of the Council of Gorges's Province in Maine, and continued in that part of the country the reft of his life. He fucceeded in 1643, by the will of Capt. Thomas Cammock, to his patent at Black Point, and foon after married his widow. He is afterwards Deputy-Governor of the Province; and until 1676, when the Indians attacked and compelled him to furrender his fort, he was, fays Mr. Willis, — whofe valuable papers are cited below, — one of the moft active

A

and influential men in it;" holding, "during all the changes of proprietorſhip and government, the moſt important offices." He is then a magiſtrate of the Duke of York's Province of Cornwall, and, as late as 1680, a reſident of Pemaquid; when he is ſpoken of, in a letter of Gov. Andros to the commander of the fort at Pemaquid, as one "whom I would have you uſe with all fitting reſpeᵗᵗ, conſidering what he hath been and his age." He is living in 1682; but had died before the 10th of May, 1683,¹ leaving no deſcendants. ²

Notwithſtanding the evidence, above afforded, of the ſocial poſition of the family of which Henry and John Joſſelyn were members, the preſent writer failed in tracing it, doubtleſs from not knowing in which county it had its principal ſeat. In this uncertainty, it occurred to him to make application to the eminent Engliſh antiquary, — the Rev. Joſeph Hunter, Vice-Preſident of the Society of Antiquaries of London, — to whom he was indebted for former kind attentions; and was favored by this gentleman with ſuch direᵗᵗions as left nothing to be deſired. "The Joſſlines," writes Mr. Hunter ("the name is written in ſome variety of ortho-

---

¹ Willis, in N. E. Geneal. Register, vol. ii. p. 204; and New Series of the same, vol. i. p. 31. Williamson, Hist. of Maine, vol. i. p. 682.

² Dr. T. W. Harris, in N. E. Geneal. Register, vol. ii. p. 306, has correᵗᵗed the mistake of Williamson and other writers as to Henry Josselyn of Scituate's being of kin to Mr. Josselyn of Black Point; and Mr. Willis, who had adopted the same error in his first paper, already cited, now admits, in his second, that there is not "any evidence that" the proprietor of Black Point "left any children, or ever had any."

graphies, and now more ufually Joceline), are quite one
of the old ariftocratic families of England, having feveral knights in the early generations; being admitted
into the order of baronets, and fubfequently into the
peerage. . . . Their main fettlement was in Hertford-
fhire, at or near the town of Sabridgeworth; and accounts of them may be read in the hiftories — of which
Chauncy's, Salmon's, and Clutterbuck's are the chief—
of that county. But a fuller and better account is to
be found in the 'Peerage of Ireland,' by Mr. Lodge,
keeper of the records in the Birmingham Tower, Dub-
lin: 4 vols. 8vo, 1754."[1]

According to Lodge, the family begins with a Sir
Egidius, who paffed into England in the time of Edward the Confeffor, and was defcended from "Carolus
Magnus, King of France, with more certainty than the
houfes of Lorraine and Guife." Of this Sir Egidius was
Sir Gilbert de Jocelyn, who accompanied the Conqueror,
and had Gilbert — called St. Gilbert, being canonized by
Pope Innocent III. in 1202 — and Geoffry. To this Geoffry is traced back John Jocelyn, living in 1226; who married Catherine, fecond daughter and co-heir to Sir Thomas
Battell, and had Thomas, who married Maud, daughter
and co-heirefs of Sir John Hide, of Hide Hall in Sabridgeworth, county of Hertford, Knt., by his wife Elizabeth, daughter of John Sudeley, Baron Sudeley, in the
county of Gloucefter. He had Thomas Jocelyn, Efq., who

---

[1] Letter of Rev. J. Hunter, 12th April, 1859.

married Joan, daughter of John Blunt, and had Ralph, who married Maud, daughter of Sir John Sutton *alias* Dudley, and had Geoffry of Hide Hall, 1312. Geoffry married Margaret, daughter of Robert Rokell or Rochill, and had Ralph, who married Margaret, daughter and heir to John Patmer, Esq., and had Geoffry (died 1425), who married Catherine, daughter and heir to Sir Thomas Bray, and had four fons and two daughters. Of thefe, the eldeft was Thomas Jocelyn, Efq., living in the reign of Edward IV., who married Alice, daughter of Lewis Duke of Dukes in Effex, Efq., by his wife Anne, daughter of John Cotton, Efq., and had iffue George, his heir, called Jocelyn the Courtier, who married Maud, daughter and heir to Edmond Bardolph, — Lord Bardolph, — and had one daughter and three fons. John Jocelyn, Efq., — "auditor of the augmentations, upon the diffolution of the abbeys by King Henry VIII.," — was fon and heir to the laft-mentioned George, and married Philippa, daughter of William Bradbury, of Littlebury in Effex; by whom he had Sir Thomas, of Hide Hall, — created a Knight of the Bath at the coronation of King Edward VI., — who married Dorothy, daughter of Sir Geoffry Gales or Gates, Knt., and had iffue;[1] one daughter marrying Roger Harlakenden, of Carnarthen in Kent, Efq.; and the fifth fon being Henry Jocelyn, Efq., who married Anne, daughter

---

[1] See also a Pedigree of Joselyne from the Visitation of Hertfordshire in 1614, furnished by Mr. S.G. Drake to the New-England Genealogical Register, vol. xiv. p. 16. This is probably one of the sources from which Lodge's account was derived.

and heir to Humphrey Torrell, otherwife Tyrrell, of Torrell's Hall in Effex, — became seated there, and had fix
fons and fix daughters. The fecond fon of this family was
Sir Thomas Jocelyn (father to our author), who was twice
married. His firft wife was Dorothy, daughter of John
Frank, Efq.; by whom he had fix fons and five daughters, — Torrell, born 28th May, 1690; Henry, and Henry,
both died infants; Thomas, who died without iffue, in
1635, at Bergen op Zoom; Edward, who, by a lady of
Georgia, had a daughter Dorothy, and died at Smyrna in
1648; Benjamin, born 19th May, 1602; Anne, married to
William Mildmay, Efq., by whom fhe had Robert, John,
Anne, and Elizabeth; Dorothy, married to John Brewfter,
Efq., and left no iffue; Elizabeth, married to Francis Neile,
Efq., and had Francis, John, and Mary; Frances, born
26th March, 1600, and married Rev. Clement Vincent;
and Mary, died unmarried. The fecond wife of Sir
Thomas Jocelyn was Theodora, daughter to Edmond
Cooke, of Mount Mafchall in Kent, Efq.; and by her he
had Henry, John, Theodora, and Thomazine. Torrell, the
eldeft fon, married, firft, Elizabeth, daughter of Sir Richard Brooke of Chefhire, — heir to her grandfather (by the
mother), Dr. Chaderton, Bifhop of Lincoln, — by whom
he had a daughter, Theodora, married to Samuel Fortrie,
Efq.,[1] to whom our author dedicates the prefent volume,
with acknowledgment of the "bounty" of his "honored
friend and kinfman."

---

[1] Lodge, Peerage of Ireland, vol. iii. p. 65, and *ante*.

The principal line of the family was continued by Richard, heir to Sir Thomas of Hide Hall; the faid Richard
being brother to our author, John Joffelyn's grandfather.
In 1665, Sir Robert Jocelyn of Hide Hall was advanced
to the dignity of baronet. The fifth fon of this Sir Robert
was Thomas; whofe fon, Robert Jocelyn, Efq., was bred
to the law; was Solicitor-General and Attorney-General
and Lord High Chancellor of. Ireland; and created, in
1743, Baron Newport of Newport, and Vifcount Jocelyn
in 1755. Robert, fon and fucceffor of this nobleman, was
created, in 1771, Earl of Roden, of High Roding, County
of Tipperary; and was anceftor to the prefent Lord
Roden.[1]

Our author, John Joffelyn, made his firft voyage to New
England in 1638; arriving in Bofton Harbor the 3d of
July, and remaining with his brother at Black Point till the
10th of October of the following year. While at Bofton,
he paid his refpects to the Governor and to Mr. Cotton,
being the bearer to the latter of fome poetical pieces from
the poet Quarles; and, as he fays, "being civilly treated
by all I had occafion to converfe with." In the account
of his firft voyage, there is no appearance of that diflike to
the Maffachufetts government and people which is obferv-
able in the narrative of the fecond, and may there not
unfairly be connected with his brother's political and religious differences with Maffachufetts.[2] His fecond voyage

[1] Lodge, *ubi supra*. Annual Register, 1771, p. 174.
[2] But there is no doubt that the author was himself as far from sharing in the
serious English thought of the Puritans of Massachusetts Bay as he was from

was made in 1663. He arrived at Nantasket the 27th of July, and foon proceeded to his brother's plantation, where he tells us he ftaid eight years, and got together the matter of the book before us. This was firft printed in 1672, but occurs alfo with later dates. It was followed, in 1674, by " An Account of Two Voyages to New England; wherein you have the Setting-out of a fhip, with the Charges; the

---

joining in their evangelical faith. Yet there is hardly more than one place in either of his books (Voyages, pp. 180-2) where this is offensively brought forward. It is worthy of remark, however, that Josselyn's family, in England, was attached rather to the Puritan side. "His family connections," says Mr. Hunter, in the letter already referred to, "appear to have been adherents to the cause of the Parliament; particularly the Harlakendens, in whose regiment a Jocelyn, named Ralph, was a chaplain." Nor is this all. "In the year 1663," continues the learned authority just cited, "there was a slight insurrectionary movement in the North; which was easily put down by the government, and the leaders executed. In a manuscript list of persons who were either openly engaged, or who were vehemently suspected of being favorers of the design, I find in the latter class the name of Capt. John Jossline." This plot was not discovered till January, 1664; and our John Josselyn "departed from London," as he says at page one of this volume, "upon an invitation of my only brother," the 28th of May of the year previous. But, if it be possible that our author was the person intended in the manuscript list as one strongly suspected of being engaged in a design against the Royal Government, the evident uncertainty of this is too great to permit us to discredit his own exposure of his political leanings, — as in the Voyages, p. 197, where. speaking of Sir F. Gorges, he says, "And, when he was between three and fourscore years of age, did personally engage in our royal martyr's service, and particularly in the siege of Bristow; and was plundered and imprisoned several times, by reason whereof he was discountenanced by the pretended Commissioners for Forraign Plantations," and so forth, — or in the face of another passage to be quoted further on, in which he acknowledges "the bounty of his royal sovereignness," to question the sincerity — which there is nothing in either of his books to throw doubt upon — of his general adhesion to the Royalist side. "The family in Hertfordshire," says Mr. Hunter, "were nonconformists; but the spirit of nonconformity seems to have spent itself at the death of Sir Strange Jocelyn, the second baronet, who died in 1734. But we may trace the Puritan influence in the present Earl of Roden, who is a conspicuous member of the religious body in England called the Evangelical." — Ms. ut sup.

Prices of all Neceſſaries for furniſhing a Planter and his Family at his firſt Coming; a Defcription of the Country, Natives, and Creatures; the Government of the Countrey as it is now poſſeſſed by the Engliſh, &c.   A large Chronological Table of the moſt Remarkable Paſſages, from the firſt Difcovering of the Continent of America to the Year 1673.". 12mo, pp. 279.   Reprinted in the third volume oi the Third Series of the Collections of the Hiſtorical Society; which edition is quoted here.   A large part of the " Voyages " is taken up with obfervations relating to natural hiſtory; and it is quite likely that the author tried in this fecond work to fupply fome of the defects of his " Rarities."   Compare efpecially the accounts of beaſts of the earth, of birds, and of fiſhes; each of which is better done in the " Voyages."

Joſſelyn was, it appears, a man of polite reading.   He quotes Lucan, Pliny, and Du Bartas; he has Latin and Italian proverbs; he is acquainted with the writings of Mr. Perkins, that famous divine; with Van Helmont; with Sandys's " Travels," and Capt. John Smith's.   His curiofity in picking up " excellent medecines " points to an acquaintance with phyfic; of his practifing which, there occur, indeed (pp. 48, 58, 63), feveral inſtances.[1]   Nor is

---

1 And see the Voyages, p, 187, for an account of a " Barbarie-Moor under cure " of the author, when he " perceived that the Moor had one skin more than Englishmen.   The skin that is basted to the flesh is bloudy, and of the same Azure colour with the veins, but deeper than the colour of our Europeans' veins. Over this is an other skin, of a tawny colour, and upon that [the] *Epidermis*, or *Cuticula*, — the flower of the skin, which is that Snake's cast; and this is tawny also.   The colour of the blew skin mingling with the tawny, makes them appear

he, by any means, uninterefted in prefcriptions for the kitchen; as fee his elaborate *recipe* for cooking eels (Voyages, p. 111), and alfo that (*ibid.*, p. 190) for a compound liquor "that exceeds *paffada*, the Nectar of the country;" which is made, he tells us, of "Syder, Maligo-Raifons, Milk, and Syrup of Clove-Gilliflowers." But his curiofity in natural hiftory, and efpecially in botany, is his chief merit; and this now gives almoft all the value that is left to his books.[1] William Wood, the author of "New-England's Profpect" (London, 1634[2]), was a better obferver, generally, than Joffelyn; but the latter makes up for his other fhort-comings by the particularity of his botanical information.

The "Voyages" was Joffelyn's laft appearance in print. He was already advanced in years, and alludes to this at page 69 of the prefent book, where he fays he fhall refer the further inveftigation of a curious plant — of which a neighbor, "wandering in the woods to find out his ftrayed cattle," had brought him a fragment — "to thofe that are younger, and better able to undergo the pains and trouble of finding it out." "Henceforth," he declares in his "Voyages," p. 151, "you are to expect no more Relations

---

black." Dr. Mitchell, the botanist of Virginia, has a paper upon the same topic, — the cause of the negro's color, — in the Philosophical Transactions; but this appears less in accordance with more recent researches (Prichard, Nat. Hist. of Man, p. 81) than Josselyn's observations.

[1] "His book is a curiosity, sometimes worth examining, but seldom to be implicitly relied on." — *Savage*, in Winthrop, N. E., vol. i. p. 267, note.

[2] Reprinted, the third edition, with an introductory essay and some notes; Boston, 1764, — the edition made use of in these notes.

from me. I am now return'd into my Native Countrey; and, by the providence of the Almighty and the bounty of my Royal Soveraigness, am difpofed to a holy quiet of ftudy and meditation for the good of my foul; and being bleffed with a tranfmentitation or change of mind, and weaned from the world, may take up for my word, *non eft mortale quod opto.*"

We may fuppofe that a rude acquaintance with the more common or important animals of a new country will commence with the difcovery of it. Thus the beginning of European knowledge of the marine animals of America goes back, doubtlefs, to the earlieft fifheries of Newfoundland; and thefe began almoft immediately after the difcovery of the continent. Game and peltry were alfo likely to come to the knowledge of the earlieft adventurers; and fcattered among thefe, from the firft, were doubtlefs men capable of regarding the world of new objeéts around them with an intelligent, if not a literate eye. Defcriptions in this way, and fpecimens, at length reached Europe, and became known to the learned there — to Gefner, Clufius, and Aldrovandus — from as early as the middle of the fixteenth century. Without being naturalifts, fuch obfervers as Heriot in Virginia (1585–6) and Wood in Maffachufetts (1634) could give valuable accounts of what they faw; and more, it may well be, was due to the Chriftian miffionaries, who accompanied or followed the adventurers, for the converfion of the heathen. Gabriel Sagard was one of thefe miffionaries, a *recollet* or reformed Francifcan monk, who went from Paris to

Canada in 1624, and fpent two years in the country of the Hurons; publifhing his "Grand Voyage du Pays des Hurons" in 1632, and enlarging it in 1636 to "Hiftoire du Canada et Voyages que les Freres Mineurs recollets y ont faits pour la Converfion des Infidelles," &c., in four books; of which the third treats of natural hiftory,[1] and is cited by Meffrs. Audubon and Bachmann (Vivip. Quadrupeds of N.A., *paffim*) for a good part of our more common and noticeable *Mammalia*. Something confiderable thus got to be known of marine animals of all forts, and of quadrupeds. But it was much longer before our birds — if we except a very few, as the blue-jay and the turkey — came to the fcientific knowledge of Europeans; and this remark is, as might be expected, at leaft equally true of our reptiles.

Quite as accidental, doubtlefs, was the beginning of European acquaintance with our plants. There are, indeed, traces of the knowledge of a few at a very early period. Dalechamp, Clufius, Lobel, and Alpinus — all authors of the fixteenth century — muft be cited occafionally in any complete fynonymy of our *Flora*. The Indian-corn, the fide-faddle flower (*Sarracenia purpurea* and *S. flava*), the columbine, the common milk-weed (*Afclepias Cornuti*), the everlafting (*Antennaria margaritacea*), and the *Arbor vitæ*, were known to the juft-mentioned botanifts before 1600. *Sarracenia flava* was fent either from Virginia, or poffibly from fome Spanifh monk

---

[1] Biographie Universelle, *in loco.*

in Florida. Clufius's figure of our well-known northern *S. purpurca* — of which he gives, however, only the leaves and bafe of the ftem (*Clus. Hift. Pl., cit.* Gerard *a* Johnfon) — was derived from a fpecimen furnifhed to him by one Mr. Claude Gonier, apothecary at Paris, who him-felf had it from Lifbon; whither we may fuppofe it was carried by fome fifherman from the Newfoundland coaft. The evening primrofe (*Œnothcra bicnnis*) was known in Europe, according to Linnæus, as early as 1614. *Polygo-num fagittatum* and *arifolium* (tear-thumb) were figured by De Laet, probably from New-York fpecimens, in his "Novus Orbis," 1633. Johnfon's edition of Gerard's "Herbal" (1636) — which was poffibly our author's manu-al in the ftudy of New-England plants — contains fome dozen North-American fpecies, furnifhed often from the garden of Mr. John Tradefcant, who had other plants from "Virginia" befide the elegant one which bears his name; and John Parkinfon — whofe "Theatrum Botanicum" (1640) is declared by Tournefort to embrace a larger number of fpecies than any work which had gone before it — defcribes, efpecially from Cornuti, a ftill larger num-ber. But the firft treatife efpecially concerned with North-American plants was that of the French author juft mentioned; which, on feveral accounts, deferves particu-lar attention.

John Robin — "fecond to none," fays Tournefort, "in the knowledge and cultivation of plants" — was placed in charge of the Royal Botanical Garden at Paris, about the year 1570; and Vefpafian Robin, "a moft diligent botanift," followed, in fimilar conneftion[1] with the larger garden founded by Lewis the Thirteenth. Both are faid to have affifted the writer whofe book we are to notice; but efpecially the latter,[2] who, there is little doubt, deferves credit for all the American fpecies defcribed in it.

The hiftory of Canadian and other new plants — " Canadenfium Plantarum, aliarumque nondum editarum Hiftoria " of Jacobus Cornuti, Doftor of Medicine, of Paris — was printed in that city (pp. 238) in 1635, under the patronage juft mentioned; and contains accounts, accompanied, in every cafe but one, with figures on copper, of thirty-feven of our plants; of which the meadow-rue is known to botanifts as *Thalictrum Cornuti;* and the common milkweed, as *Asclepias Cornuti.* Though himself not eminent as a botanift,[3] the work of Cornuti was valua-

[1] He is called *Botanicus Regius* by Cornuti, p. 22; and the same title is given to both the Robins, in the printed catalogue of plants cultivated by them. Tournefort indicates the office of Vespasian Robin, at the new Botanic Garden, as follows: " *Brossæus* . . . primus Horti præfeɛtus, studiosis plantas indigitandi numeri præposuit Vespasianum Robinum diligentissimum Botanicum." — *Inst. Rei Herb.,* vol. i. p. 48. And the recent writer in the Biographie Universelle, says, more expressly, that the royal *ordonnance* establishing the garden names Vespasian Robin "sub-demonstrator" of botany, with a stipend of two hundred francs yearly. According to this writer, the two Robins were not, as has been said. father and son, but brothers; and Vespasian the elder. This one must have reached a great age, as the celebrated Morrison, who visited France in 1640, and remained there twelve years, calls himself his disciple. — *Biog. Universelle, in loco.*

[2] Tournefort, *ubi supra.*

[3] Cornuti autem parum fuit in plantarum cognitione versatus, ut manifestum est ex ineptis appellationibus quibus utitur in Enchiridio Botanico Parisiensi, et descriptionibus speciosis·ab Herbariorum stylo tamen alienis. — *Tournef. Inst.,* vol. i. p. 43. Compare, as to the botanical merits of Cornuti, the writer in Biographie Universelle, who says that Cornuti's terminology, to which Tournefort

ble for its elegant prefentation of much that was new; and
it will always deferve honorable remembrance in the hiftory of our *Flora*. There are feveral paffages of it — as
at pp. 5 and 7, and in the account of the two baneberries
at p. 76, where we read, "Opacis et fylveftribus locis in
eadem Americæ parte frequentiffimum eft geminum genus" — which look a little like a proper botanical collec-
tor's notes on his fpecimens; and thefe fpecimens, and the
others from the fame region, may well have been refults
of the herborizing of that worthy Francifcan miffionary,
whofe early obfervations on the natural hiftory of Canada
have been mentioned already above.   Nor were the
North-American plants poffeffed by Cornuti entirely confined to this region; for he fpeaks at the end (p. 214) of
his having received a root, *ex notha Anglia*, as he ftrangely
calls it, known, it appears, by the name of *Serpentaria*, or,
in the vernacular, *Snaqroel*, — a fure remedy for the bite
of a huge and moft pernicious ferpent *in notha Anglia*, —
which was no doubt the fnake-root fo famous once as a
cure for the bite of a rattlefnake, and one of the numerous
varieties of *Nabalus albus* (L.) Hook., if not, as Purfh
fuppofed, what is now the *var. Serpentaria*, Gray.   But
fome view of the fcantinefs of fcientific knowledge of our
Flora, near forty years after Cornuti, may be had by reckoning the number of fpecies for which Bauhin's "Pinax"

---

took exception, was that of Lobel; and farther, that the catalogue — Enchiridium
Botanicum Parisiense — which is annexed to Cornuti's larger work, is in several
refpects creditable to him. — *Biog. Univ., in loco.*

and "Prodromus" (1671) are cited by Linnæus in the "Species Plantarum." Moſt of them are Southern plants; and the few decidedly Northern ones which meet us — as *Cornus Canadenſis, Uvularia perfoliata, Trillium erectum, Arum triphyllum,* and *Adiantum pedatum* — are all indicated, by Bauhin's phraſe, as from Brazil!

We have nothing illuſtrating the *Flora* of New England from Cornuti till Joſſelyn. In Virginia, Mr. John Baniſter, a correſpondent of Ray's, began to botanize probably not long after the middle of the ſeventeenth century. He was ſucceeded by ſeveral eminent names; as Mark Catesby, F.R.S. (born 1679), John Clayton, Eſq. (born 1685), and John Mitchell, M.D., F.R.S., — a contemporary of the other two, — who together gave to the botany of Virginia a diſtinguiſhed luſtre; as did Cadwalader Colden, Eſq. (born 1688), — a ſelection from whoſe correſpondence has been lately edited by Dr. Gray, — to that of New York; John Bartram (born 1701), "American botaniſt to his Britannic Majeſty," to that of Pennſylvania; and, ſomewhat later, Alexander Garden, M.D., F.R.S. (born 1728), to that of South Carolina. Joſſelyn himſelf is, indeed, little more than a herbaliſt; but it is enough that he gets beyond that entirely unſcientific character. He certainly botanized, and made botanical uſe of Gerard and his other authorities. The credit belongs to him of indicating ſeveral genera as new which were ſo, and peculiar to the American *Flora.* It may at leaſt be ſaid, that, at the time he wrote, there is no reaſon to ſuppoſe that any other perſon knew as much as he did of the botany of New

England. "The plants in New England," he fays in his "Voyages," p. 59, "for the variety, number, beauty, and virtues, may ftand in competition with the plants of any countrey in Europe. Johnfon hath added to Gerard's 'Herbal' three hundred, and Parkinfon. mentioneth many more. Had they been in New England, they might have found a thoufand, at leaft, never heard of nor feen by any Englifhman before."[1]   Nor did our author fail to adorn his "Rarities" with recognizable figures, as well as de-fcriptions, of fome of thefe new American plants; and

---

[1] Mention of New-England plants may be found in earlier writers than Cor-nuti or Josselyn; but what is said is now rarely available. Gosnold's expedition was in 1602; and the writer of the account of it tells us that the island upon which his party proposed to settle (Cuttyhunk, one of the Elizabeth Islands) was covered with "oaks, ashes, beech, walnut, witch-hazel, sassafrage, and cedars, with divers others of unknown names;" beside "wild pease, young sassafrage, cherry-trees, vines, eglantine, gooseberry-bushes, hawthorn, honeysuckles, with others of the like quality;" as also "strawberries, rasps, ground-nuts, alexander, surrin, tansy, &c., without count." — *Mass. Hist. Coll.*, vol. xxviii. p. 76. And so the writer of Mourt's Relation, in 1620, speaks of "sorrel, yarrow, carvel, brook-lime, liverwort, watercresses, &c., as noticed, "in winter," however, at Plymouth. — *Hist. Coll.* vol. viii. p. 221. There is much here which is true enough, though the "eglantine" of the first writer is an evident mistake, as doubtless also the "carvel" of the other; but we have no reason to suppose that either of. these passages ever had any scientific value. Josselyn, so far as his Botany goes, does not belong to this class of writers. There are important parts of his account of our plants, in which we know with certainty what he intended to tell us; and, farther, that this was worth the telling. And the credit which fairly belongs to the new *genera* of American plants, in some sort indicated by him, shall illustrate as well those other portions of his work where what he meant is a matter rather of deduction from his particulars, such as they are, in the light of his only here-and-there-cited authorities, than of plain fact. His English names — com-mon, and perhaps often indefinite, as they strike us — had more of scientific value, in botanical hands at least, when he wrote, than now; and, there is good reason to suppose, were meant to indicate that the plants intended, or in some cases the *genera* to which they belonged, were the same with those published, under the same names, by Gerard, Johnson, and Parkinson.

his arrangement is alfo creditable to his botanical knowledge. By this arrangement, his collections are diftinguifhed into —

1. " Such plants as are common with us in England."
2. " Such plants as are proper to the country."
3. " Such plants as are proper to the country, and have no name."
4. " Such plants as have fprung up fince the English planted and kept
   cattle in New England."

The laft of thefe divifions is the moft valuable part of
Joffelyn's account, as it affords the only teftimony that
there is to the firft notice among us of a number of now
naturalized weeds, which it is an interefting queftion to
feparate from the more important clafs of plants truly
indigenous in, and common to, both hemifpheres; and the
author's treatment of the latter — as indeed of the other
two lifts mentioned above — fhows that he was competent,
in a meafure, to reckon the former. This furnifhes a date,
and an early one; and there is no other till 1785, when
Dr. Manaffeh Cutler's Memoir, to be fpoken of, enables us
to limit the appearance of fome other fpecies not mentioned by Joffelyn.

There is no work of any fize or importance on New-
England plants, after Joffelyn, for the whole century which
followed. We were not, indeed, without men in diftinguifhed connection with the European fcientific world.
The moft eminent New-England family gained honors in
fcience, as well as in the conduct of affairs. John Winthrop the younger, eldeft fon of the firft Governor of
Maffachufetts, — and the "heir," fays Savage, "of all his

c

father's talents, prudence, and virtues, with a fuperior
fhare of human learning,"[1]—was himfelf the firft Governor of Connecticut, and had, in this conneĉtion, a certain fcientific pofition and reputation. "The great Mr.
Boyle, Bifhop Wilkins, with feveral other learned men,"
fays Dr. Eliot, "had propofed to leave England, and eftab-
lifh a fociety for promoting natural knowledge in the new
colony of which Mr. Winthrop, their intimate friend and
affociate, was appointed Governor. Such men were too
valuable to lofe from Great Britain; and, Charles II. having taken them under his proteĉtion, the fociety was there
eftablifhed, and obtained the title of the Royal Society of
London. . . . Mr. Winthrop fent over many fpecimens of
the produĉtions of this country, with his remarks upon
them: 'and, by an order of the Royal Society, he was in
a particular manner invited to take upon himfelf the charge
of being the chief correfpondent in the Weft, as Sir
Philiberto Vernatti was in the Eaft Indies.' 'His name,'
fays the fame writer, Dr. Cromwell Mortimer, Secretary of
the Royal Society, in his flattering dedication of the forti-
eth volume of the Philofophical Tranfaĉtions to the Governor's grandfon, 'had he put it to his writings, would
have been as univerfally known as the Boyles's, the Wilkins's, and Oldenburghs', and been handed down to us
with fimilar applaufe.'"[2] There is, in the volume of
Philofophical Tranfaĉtions for 1670, "An Extraĉt of a

[1] Winthrop's Journal, by Savage, edit. 1, vol. i. p. 64, note. See also Ban-
croft's charaĉter of the younger Winthrop, in History of the United States, vol.
ii. p. 52.
[2] Eliot, Biog. Diĉt., in loco.

Letter written by John Winthrop, Efq., Governor of Connecticut in New England, to the Publifher, concerning
fome 'Natural Curiofities of thofe Parts; efpecially a very
ftrange and curioufly-contrived Fifh, fent for the Repofitory of the Royal Society " (pp. 3); in which are mentioned, as fent, fpecimens of fcrub-oak; "bark of tree
with fir-balfam, which grows in Nova Scotia, and, as I
hear, in the more eafterly part of New England;" pods of
milk-weed, "ufed to ftuff pillows and cufhions;" and "a
branch of the tree called the cotton-tree, bearing a kind of
down, which alfo is not fit to fpin."

Fitz John Winthrop, Efq., F.R.S. (died 1707), fon of
the laft, and alfo Governor of Connecticut, is faid to have
been "famous for his philofophical" (that is, fcientific)
"knowledge."[1]   And the fecond Governor's nephew, John
Winthrop, Efq., F.R.S. (died 1747), who left this country
and paffed the latter part of his life in England, is declared
by the author of the dedication already above cited, to
have "increafed the riches of their" (the Royal Society's)
"repofitory with more than fix hundred curious fpecimens,
chiefly in the mineral kingdom; accompanied with an
accurate account of each particular."   "Since Mr. Col-
well," it is added, "the founder of the Mufeum of the
Royal Society, you have been the benefactor who has
given the moft numerous collection."   Dr. John Winthrop,
F.R.S. (died 1779), Hollifian Profeffor of Mathematics at
Cambridge, N.E., whofe important papers on aftronomical

---

[1] Eliot, Biog. Dict., *in loco.*

and other related phenomena are to be found in the Philofophical Tranfaćtions, was of another line of the fame
family.

Paul Dudley, Efq., F.R.S. (born 1675), fon of Gov.
Jofeph Dudley, and himfelf Chief Juſtice of Maſſachuſetts,
was author of feveral papers in the Philofophical Tranfaćtions; one of which is an "Account of the Poifon-wood
Tree in New-England" (vol. xxxi. p. 135); and another,
"Obfervations on fome Plants in New-England, with
Remarkable Inſtances of the Nature and Power of Vege-
tation" (vol. xxxiii. p. 129). This laſt is of only feven
pages, and of little fcientific account: though we learn
from it, that, in 1726, when Mr. Dudley wrote, the Pear-
main, Kentiſh Pippin, and Golden Ruſſetin, were eſteemed
apples here, and the Orange and Bergamot cultivated
pears;[1] that, in one town in 1721, they made three thoufand, and in another near ten thoufand barrels of cider;
and that, to fpeak of "trees of the wood," he knew of a

---

[1] Interleaved Almanacs of 1646–48, cited by Savage (Winthrop. N. E., vol. ii.
p. 332). mention "Tankard" and "Kreton" (perhaps Kirton) apples, as well as
Russetins, Pearmains, and Long-Red apples; beside "the great pears," and ap-
ricots, as grown here. In the Records of the Governor and Company of the
Massachusetts Bay (Records of Mass., vol. i. p. 24), there is an undated memorandum, "To provide to send for Newe England . . . stones of all sorts of
fruites; as peaches, plums, filberts, cherries, pear, aple, quince kernells," &c.,
which the "First General Letter of the Governor," &c., of the 17th April, 1629,
again makes mention of (ibid., p. 392); and Josselyn (Voyages, p. 189) remarks
on the "good fruit" reared from such kernels. But, if this were the only source
of our ancestors' English fruit, the names which they gave to the seedlings must
have been vague. — For other early notices of cultivated fruit-trees, see Savage
Gen. Dićt. 4. p. 258, and the same, 4. p. 621. Saml. Sewall, jun. Esq., of Brook-
line, had trees grafted with 'Drew's Russet,' and 'Golden Russet' apples, in
1724. (Gen. Reg. 16, p. 65.)

button-wood tree which meafured nine yards in girth, and made twenty-two cords of wood; and of an afh, which, at a yard from the ground, was fourteen feet eight inches in girth. He alfo expreffes an intention to treat feparately the evergreens of New England; and this treatife, which was poffibly more valuable than the one juft noticed, was in the poffeffion of Peter Collinfon, the eminent patron of horticulture, and was given by him to J. F. Gronovius; but has not, that I am aware of, appeared in print.[1]

It is likely that the early phyficians of New England gave fpecial attention to thofe fimples of the country, the virtues of which were known to the favages; and perhaps it was partly in this way that the Rev. Jared Eliot (born 1685), minifter of Killingworth in Connecticut, — who is called by Dr. Allen "the firft phyfician of his day," — is alfo defignated, both by him and by Eliot, a botanift; and by the latter, "the firft in New England." There is no doubt he was a friend of Dr. Franklin's, and a fcientific agriculturift according to the knowledge of his day; and he is faid to have introduced the white mulberry into Connecticut.[2] His Agricultural Effays went through more than one edition, but is now rare. Mr. Eliot died while our next character, the firft native New-England botanift who deferves the name, was a ftudent of Yale College.

[1] Gronov. *Fl. Virg.*, edit. 2. In Mr. Dillwyn's (unpublished) "Account of the Plants cultivated by the late Peter Collinson," from his own catalogue and other manuscripts, I find Collinson quoting Mr. Dudley's paper on Plants of New England, above mentioned; but not that on the Evergreens. — *Hortus Collins.*, p. 41.

[2] Eliot, Biog. Dict., and Allen, Amer. Biog. Dict., *in locis*.

Manaſſeh Cutler, LL.D. (born 1743), was miniſter of
the Hamlet in Ipſwich — afterwards incorporated as the
town of Hamilton — fifty-one years, and was alſo a member of the Medical Society of Maſſachuſetts. He is author
of "An Account of ſome of the Vegetable Productions
naturally growing in this part of America, botanically
arranged," which makes nearly a hundred pages of the firſt
volume of the Memoirs of the American Academy, 1785.
In the introduction to this paper, the author ſpeaks of
Canada and the Southern States having had attention
given to their productions, both by ſome of their own
inhabitants and by European naturaliſts; while "that ex-
tenſive tract of country which lies between them, includ-
ing ſeveral degrees of latitude, and exceedingly diverſified
in its ſurface and ſoil, ſeems ſtill to remain unexplored."
He attributes the neglect, in part, to this, — "that botany
has never been taught in any of our colleges," but princi-
pally to the prevalent opinion of its unprofitableness in
common life. The latter error he combats with the then
important obſervation, that, "though all the medicinal
properties and economical uſes of plants are not diſcovera-
ble from thoſe characters by which they are ſyſtematically
arranged, yet the celebrated Linnæus has found that the
virtues of plants may be, in a conſiderable degree, and
moſt ſafely, determined by their *natural* characters: for
plants of the ſame *natural* claſs are in some meaſure ſimi-
lar; thoſe of the ſame *natural* order have a ſtill nearer
affinity; and thoſe of the ſame genus have very ſeldom
been found to differ in their medical virtues" (p. 397).

This fhows, perhaps, that Dr. Cutler appreciated (for the *Italics* in the juft-quoted paffage are his own) that adumbration of a natural fyftem which was afforded or fuggefted by the artificial; and his inftances — the *Graminea*, the *Borraginacea*, the *Umbellifera*, the *Labiata*, the *Crucifera*, the *Malvacea*, the *Compofita*, &c.; though thefe are cited under the divifions, not of the natural, but of the fexual fyftem — are ftill more to the point. There are other obfervations of intereft; and the fuggeftion is made, that perfons fhould collect the plants of their diftricts, and fend them from time to time to the Academy.

Dr. Cutler was thus, poffibly, the firft to fuggeft a botanical chair in our colleges, and a general *herbarium* to illuftrate the *Flora* of New England; and perhaps it was this laft which led him to propofe a ftill more important undertaking. "It has long been my intention," he fays in a letter to Prof. Swartz, of Upfal, dated 15th October, 1802, "to publifh a botanical work, comprifing the plants of the northern and eaftern States; and [I] have been collecting materials for that purpofe. But numerous avocations, and a variety of other engagements, has occafioned delay. It is, however, ftill my intention, if my health permits, to do it. But, at this time, far lefs than in years paft, there is very little encouragement given here to publications of this kind."[1]

About three hundred and feventy plants are indicated in the publifhed "Account" of Dr. Cutler. It was not to be

---

[1] Mss. Cutler, *penes me*.

expected, that, in this beginning, numerous miftakes fhould not be made. It could not poffibly have been otherwife. There is ftill evidence enough of the author's genius, which perhaps needed only opportunity and encouragement to anticipate a part of what botany now owes to a Nuttall, a Torrey, and a Gray. The "Account" was favorably received by other botanifts of the time, both in this country and abroad. In a letter of Muhlenberg to Cutler, dated 9th February, 1791, the former fays, "Not till a few months ago, I was favored with the firft volume of the Memoirs of the American Academy of Arts and Sciences, printed at Bofton, 1785. Amongft other valuable pieces, I found your 'Account of Indigenous Vegetables, botanically arranged;' with which I was infinitely pleafed, as this was the firft work that gives a fyftematical account of New-England plants. Being a great friend to botany, and having ftudied it in my leifure-hours upwards of fourteen years in Pennfylvania, I know the difficulty of arranging the American plants according to the Linnean fyftem; and I was always eager to hear of fome gentleman engaged in fimilar refearches, that, by joining hands, we might do fomething towards enlarging American Botany. . . . This is the reafon why I intrude upon your leifure-hours, and crave for your acquaintance and friendfhip."[1] Drs. Withering and Stokes, of England, were other correfpondents of Cutler, and furnifhed him with important obfervations upon his printed Memoir, befides fpecimens;

---

[1] Mss. Cutler, *penes me.*

as did alfo Swartz, and, it appears, Payfhull of Sweden. Dr. Stokes followed up his various fuggeftions for
the improvement of the Memoir, by propofing to ded-
icate a plant, which he took to be new, to its author.
"A plant," he fays, "like a woolly heath, and which I
wifhed to call *Cutleria ericoides*, turns out to be *Hudfonia ericoides*. I hope, however, your herborizations may
furnifh a new genus for you, not likely to be difturbed."
— *Letters of Stokes to Cutler*, from "Feb. 14, '91, to Aug.
17, '93."[1]

But Dr. Cutler's printed memoir on the plants of New
England is much furpaffed in intereft by his manufcript
volumes of defcriptions, ftill extant. Thefe manufcript
volumes commence with "Book I., 1783," and continue, fo
far as I have feen them, to 1804. The late Mr. Oakes
poffeffed fix of thefe books; and two were given to me by
my valued friend, the late Dr. T. W. Harris. They are
generally entitled, "Defcriptions and Notes on American
Indigenous Plants," and contain a vaft number of obfervations and analyfes, fometimes accompanied by pen-and-ink
sketches. This was evidently the material accumulated
for the author's *Flora* above mentioned; and the following
extracts will ferve to fhow that he was in many refpects
qualified to undertake fuch a work. Thus, in defcribing
the feveral hickories, he points out thofe differences from
Juglans, upon which Nuttall afterwards conftituted his

---

[1] Mss. Cutler, *penes me.*

D

genus *Carya*. Again, in the fame volume, — that for
1789, — there is a *N. Gen. Anonymos*, minutely defcribed
in feveral pages, which is no other than *Thefium umbella-
tum*, L., afterwards diftinguifhed by Nuttall as his genus
Comandra. Again, under *Anonymos, Yellow-Sandbind*,
there is a full defcription of what Nuttall after named
Hudfonia tomentofa. The fame volume fhows that the
author had anticipated Prof. Gray in referring *Orchis
fimbriata*, as it was called by Purfh and other botanifts, to
O. pfychodes, L.; and the remark is alfo made that *O.
lacera* Michx., — which Muhlenberg and our other writers
had miftakenly referred to *O. pfychodes*, till Dr. Gray corrected the error, — muft be a new fpecies," which it then
certainly was. Again, there is another *Anomolos* defcribed
at length, which is the fame afterwards conftituted by
Nuttall his genus *Microftylis*. So *Campanula humida*
(Cutler mfs.) is what Purfh defignated, long after, *C.
aparinoides*. Again, in another volume (for 1800), he
anticipates Purfh by propofing for our water-fhield the
name *Brafenia ovalifolia;* and, in yet another, he is before
Bigelow in defcribing as a new fpecies what the latter,
many years later, publifhed as *Prunus obovata*. This may
fuffice to indicate the merits of the botanift of Ipfwich
Hamlet. A little fhrub-willow, with clean, fhining leaves,
and modeft catkins, — inhabiting, almoft everywhere, the
alpine regions of the White Mountains, and gathered by
him there, before any other botanift had penetrated thofe
folitudes, — ftill reminds us of his name, which deferves to
be remembered by his countrymen.

After Cutler, there appeared nothing of importance[1] on our botany, till the prefent elder fchool of New-England botanifts — a fchool characterized by the names of an Oakes, a Boott, and an Emerfon — was founded, now more than forty years ago, by the claffical *Florula* of Bigelow.

---

[1] The late Dr. Waterhouse, Professor of Medicine at Cambridge, read lectures on Natural History to his classes as early as 1788, and published the botanical part of these lectures in the Monthly Anthology, 1804-8; reprinting this in 1811, with the title of the Botanist (Boston, 8vo, pp. 228). In the preface to this volume, the author's are claimed to have been the first public lectures on Natural History given in the United States. The Massachusetts Professorship of Botany and Entomology was founded in 1805, and the Botanical Garden in 1807; but the eminent naturalist who first filled the chair left little behind him to bear witness to his acknowledged "learning and genius." — *Quincy*, *Hist. Harv. Univ.*, vol. ii. p. 330. The studies of Peck were not, however, confined to the *Fauna* and *Flora* of New England; and his distinguished successors in the lecture-room and the botanical garden — Mr. Nuttall, the late Dr. Harris, and Professor Gray — may be said to have maintained a like general, rather than local character, in the entomological and botanical investigations pursued at the University.

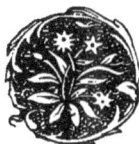

New-Englands

RARITIES
Difcovered :

I N

Birds, Beafts, Fifhes, Serpents, and *Plants*
of that Country.

Together with

The *Phyfical* and *Chyrurgical* REMEDIES wherewith the *Natives* conftantly ufe to Cure their
DISTEMPERS, WOUNDS, and SORES.

A L S O

A perfect *Defcription* of an *Indian SQUA*, in all
her Bravery; with a POEM not improperly
conferr'd upon her.

LASTLY

A CHRONOLOGICAL TABLE
of the moft remarkable Paffages in that Country
amongft the ENGLISH.

Iluftrated with CUTS.

By *JOHN JOSSELYN*, Gent.

London, Printed for *G. Widdowes* at the
Green Dragon in St. *Pauls* Church yard, 1672.

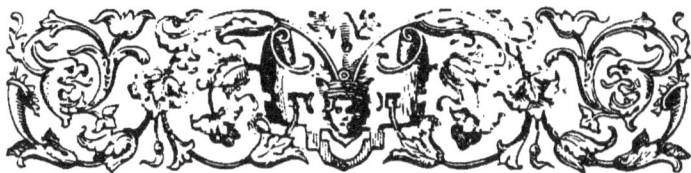

To the highly obliging,

His Honoured Friend and Kinsman,

SAMUEL FORTREY Efq;

S I R,

*I*T *was by your affiftance (enabling me) that I com-
menc'd a Voyage into thofe remote parts of the World
(known to us by the painful Difcovery of that memorable
Gentleman Sir* Fran. Drake.) *Your bounty then and
formerly hath engaged a retribution of my Gratitude,
and not knowing how to teftifie the fame unto you other-
wayes, I have (although with fome reluctancy) adven-
tured to obtrude upon you thefe rude and indigefted
Eight Years Obfervations, wherein whether I fhall more
fhame my felf or injure your accurate Judgment and
better Employment in the perufal, is a queftion.*

We read of Kings and Gods that kindly took
A Pitcher fill'd with Water from the Brook.

The Contemplation whereof (well knowing your noble and generous Difpofition) hath confirm'd in me the hope that you will pardon my prefumption, and accept the tender of the fruits of my Travel after this homely manner, and my felf as,

Sir,

Your highly obliged,

&

moft humble Servant,

John Joffelyn.

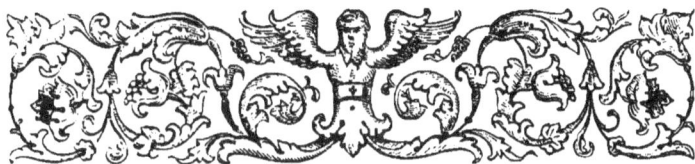

New-Englands

RARITIES

Difcovered.

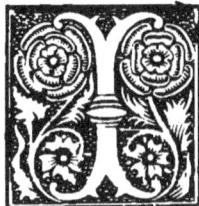

IN the year of our Lord 1663. *May* 28. upon an Invitation from my only Brother, I departed from *London*, and arrived at *Bofton*, the chief Town in the *Maffachu-fetts*, a Colony of *Englifhmen* in *New-England*, the 28*th* of *July* following.

Bofton (whofe longitude is 315 deg. and 42 deg. 30 min. of North Latitude) is built on the South-weft fide of a Bay large enough for the Anchorage of 500 Sail of Ships, the Buildings are handfome, joyning one to the other as in *London*, with many large ftreets, moft of them paved with pebble ftone, in the high ftreet towards the Common, there are fair buildings, fome of ftone, and at the Eaft End of the [2] Town one amongft the reft, built by the Shore by Mr. *Gibs*, a Merchant, being a ftately Edifice, which it is thought will ftand him in little lefs

E

than 3000 *l.* before it be fully finifhed.[1] The Town is
not divided into Parifhes, yet they have three fair Meeting-
houfes or Churches, which hardly fuffice to receive the
Inhabitants and Strangers that come in from all parts.[2]

Having refrefhed my felf here for fome time, and oppor-
tunely lighting upon a paffage in a Bark belonging to a
Friend of my Brothers, and bound to the Eaftward, I put
to sea again, and on the Fifteenth of *Auguft,* I arrived at
Black-point, otherwife called *Scarborow,* the habitation of
my beloved Brother,[3] being about an hundred leagues to the

· [1] This house was one Mr. Robert Gibbs's "of an ancient family in Devon-
shire," says Farmer (Geneal. Reg., p. 120); and it stood on Fort Hill, the way
leading to it becoming afterwards known as Gibbs's Lane, and a wharf at the
waterside, belonging to the property, as Gibbs's Wharf. Mr. W. B. Trask, who
obligingly examined for me the early deeds concerning this estate in Suffolk
Registry, furnishes a *memorandum,* that on the 6th June, 1671, Robert Gibbs of
Boston, merchant, conveys to Edward and Elisha Hutchinson, in trust, for Elizabeth, wife of said Robert, during her life, and after her decease to such child or
children as he shall have by her, his land and house on Fort Hill, with warehouse
on wharf, 'which land was formerly my grandfather, Henry Webb's.' The wife
of said Robert Gibbs was daughter to Jacob Sheafe by Margaret, daughter to
Henry Webb, mercer. Sampson Sheafe, a Provincial councillor of New Hampshire,
and the ancestor of a family of long standing there, married another daughter of
Jacob Sheafe. Mr. Gibbs was father to the Rev. Henry Gibbs, minister of Watertown, and had other children; and the family continues to this day.

[2] Compare the author's Voyages, pp. 19, 161, 173, for other notices of Boston,
and as to the first of these, which represents the town (in 1638) as "rather a
village, . . . there being not above twenty or thirty houses," see the note in
Savage's Winthrop, edit. 1, vol. i. p. 267.

[3] Mr. Henry Josselyn was probably living at Black Point in 1638, when his
brother first visited it (Voyages, p. 20). It was then the estate (by grant from
the council at Plymouth) and residence of Captain Thomas Cammock; but he,
dying in 1643, bequeathed it, except five hundred acres which were reserved to his
wife, to Josselyn, who, marrying the widow, succeeded to the whole property,
which was described as containing fifteen hundred acres (Willis *infra*), but is
called by Sullivan five thousand (History of Maine, p. 128). In 1658, this and
other adjoining tracts were erected into a town by Massachusetts, under the name

Eaftward of *Bofton*; here I refided eight years, and made it my bufinefs to difcover all along the Natural, Phyfical, and Chyrurgical Rarities of this New-found World.

New-England is faid to begin at 40 and to end at 46 of Northerly Latitude, that is from *de la Ware* Bay to *New-found-Land*.

The Sea Coafts are accounted wholfomeft, the Eaft and South Winds coming [3] from Sea produceth warm weather, the Northweft coming over land caufeth extremity of Cold, and many times ftrikes the Inhabitants both *Englifh* and *Indian* with that fad Difeafe called there the Plague of the back, but with us *Empiema*.[1]

The Country generally is Rocky and Mountanous, and extremely overgrown with wood, yet here and there beautified with large rich Valleys, wherein are Lakes ten, twenty, yea fixty miles in compafs, out of which our great Rivers have their Beginnings.[2]

Fourfcore miles (upon a direct line) to the Northweft of *Scarborow*, a Ridge of Mountains run Northweft and

---

of Scarborough, which is thus further noticed by our author in his Voyages, p. 201, as " the town of Black Point, consisting of about fifty dwelling-houses, and a Magazine, or *Doganne*, scatteringly built. They have store of neat and horses, of sheep near upon seven or eight hundred, much arable and marsh, salt and fresh, and a corn-mill." — Comp. Williamson's Hist. of Maine, vol. i. pp. 392, 666; Willis in Geneal. Register, vol. i. p. 202.

[1] *Empyema* is a result of disease of the lungs. See Voyages, p. 121.

[2] Compare the accounts of the first appearance of the country by the Rev. Francis Higginson and Mr Thomas Graves, both well-qualified observers, in New-England's Plantation, London, 1630; reprinted in Mass. Hist. Coll., vol. i. p. 117. And see Wood's New England's Prospect, a book which our author was probably acquainted with; as compare p. 4 of Wood (edit. 1764) with the beginning of p. 3 of the Rarities, and some other places in both.

Northeaft an hundred Leagues, known by the name of the
White Mountains, upon which lieth Snow all the year, and
is a Land-mark twenty miles off at Sea.   It is rifing
ground from the Sea fhore to thefe Hills, and they are
inacceffible but by the Gullies which the diffolved Snow
hath made; in thefe Gullies grow *Saven* Bufhes, which
being taken hold of are a good help to the climbing Dif-
coverer; upon the top of the higheft of thefe Mountains
is a large Level [4] or Plain of a days journey over,
whereon nothing grows but Mofs; at the farther end of
this Plain is another Hill called the *Sugar-Loaf,* to out-
ward appearance a rude heap of maffie ftones piled one
upon another, and you may as you afcend ftep from one
ftone to another, as if you were going up a pair of ftairs,
but winding ftill about the Hill till you come to the top,
which will require half a days time, and yet it is not
above a Mile, where there is alfo a Level of about an
Acre of ground, with a pond of clear water in the midft of
it; which you may hear run down, but how it afcends is a
myftery.   From this rocky Hill you may fee the whole
Country round about; it is far above the lower Clouds,
and from hence we beheld a Vapour (like a great Pillar)
drawn up by the Sun Beams out of a great Lake or Pond
into the Air, where it was formed into a Cloud.   The
Country beyond thefe Hills Northward is daunting terrible, being full of rocky Hills, as thick as Mole-hills in a
Meadow, and cloathed with infinite thick Woods.[1]

---

[1] The earliest ascents of the White Mountains were those made by Field and
others in 1642, of which we have some account in Winthrop's Journal (by Savage,

New-England is by fome affirmed to be an Ifland,
bounded on the North with the [5] River *Canada*, (fo

---

edit. 1, vol. ii. pp. 67, 89). Darby Field, "an Irishman living about Pascata-
quack," has the honor of being the first European who set foot upon the summit
of Mount Washington. He appears at Exeter in 1639. and was at Dover in 1645,
and died there in 1649, leaving a widow, and, it is said, children (A. H. Quint,
N. E. Geneal. Reg., vol. vi. p. 38). It seems likely, from his account, that Field,
on reaching the Indian town in the Saco Valley, "at the foot of the hill" where
the "two branches of Saco river met," pursued his way up the valley either of
Rocky Branch or of Ellis River, till he gradually attained to the region of dwarf
firs, on what is known as Boott's Spur, which is between the "valley" called
Oakes's Gulf, in which the "Mount Washington" branch of the Saco has its
head, and the valley in which the Rocky Branch rises (see G. P. Bond's Map of
the White Mountains). There is no other way that shall fulfil the conditions
of the narrative except that over Boott's Spur; but of the three streams, that is,
"the two branches of Saco River," which come together at or near the probable
site of the Indian town, the Rocky Branch is the shortest, and its valley the most
ascending. Field repeated his visit, with some others, "about a month after;"
and later, in the same year, the mountains were visited by the worshipful Thomas
Gorges. Esq., Deputy-Governor, and Richard Vines, Esq., Councillor of the Province of Maine, of which Winthrop takes notice at p. 89. Whether Josselyn
went up himself. or had his account from others, does not appear. But his calling the mountains "inaccessible but by the gullies," leaves it at least supposable,
that he, or the party from which he got his information (perhaps Gorges's),
instead of gradually ascending the long ridges, or spurs, penetrated into one of
the gulfs (as they are there called), or ravines, of the eastern side; the walls of
which are exceedingly steep, and literally inaccessible in many parts, except by
the gullies. The "large level or plain of a day's journey over, whereon grows
nothing but moss," is noticed in Winthrop's account of Gorges's ascent, but not
in that of Field's; and this plain — which doubtless includes what has since been
called "Bigelow's Lawn" (lying immediately under the south-eastern side of the
summit of Mount Washington), but understood also, in Gorges's account, to ex-
tend northward as far as the "Lake of the Clouds" — furnishes another ground
for supposing that the last-mentioned explorer, or, at least, Josselyn, may have
penetrated the mountain by one of its eastern ravines; several of which head in
the great plain mentioned, while that is rather remote from what we have taken
for Field's "ridge." Our author is the only authority for the "pond of clear
water in the midst of" the top of Mount Washington; though a somewhat capa-
cious spring. which was well known there before the putting-up of the house on
the summit. may have been larger once; or he may rather have mistaken, or
misremembered, the position of the Lake of the Clouds.

called from Monfieur *Cane*) on the South with the River *Mohegan*, or *Hudfons* River, fo called becaufe he was the firft that difcovered it.[1] Some will have *America* to be an Ifland, which out of queftion muft needs be, if there be a Northeaft paffage found out into the South Sea; it contains 1152400000 Acres. The difcovery of the Northweft paffage (which lies within the River of *Canada*) was undertaken with the help of fome Proteftant *Frenchmen*, which left *Canada* and retired to *Bofton* about the year 1669. The Northeaft people of *America* i.e. *New England, &c.* are judged to be *Tartars* called *Samoades*, being alike in complexion, fhape, habit and manners, (fee the *Globe:*) Their Language is very fignificant, ufing but few words, every word having a diverfe fignification, which is expreft by their gefture; as when they hold their head of one fide the word fignifieth one thing, holding their hand up when they pronounce it fignifieth another thing. Their Speeches in their Affemblies are very gravely delivered, commonly in perfect *Hexamiter* Verfe, with great filence and attention, and anfwered again *ex tempore* after the fame manner.[2]

[6] Having given you fome fhort Notes concerning the Country in general, I fhall now enter upon the propofed Difcovery of the Natural, Phyfical, and Chyrurgical Rarities; and that I may methodically deliver them unto you,

---

[1] Compare, as to the insulation of the tract understood by Josselyn as New England, Palfrey, Hist. N. E., vol. i. pp. 1, 2, and note, and the accompanying map.

[2] See the author's larger account of the natives in his Voyages, pp. 123-150.

I fhall caft them into this form: 1. Birds. 2. Beafts. 3. Fifhes. 4. Serpents and Infects. 5. Plants, of thefe, 1. fuch Plants as are common with us, 2. of fuch Plants as are proper to the country, 3. of fuch Plants as are proper to the Country and have no name known to us, 4. of fuch Plants as have fprung up fince the *Englifh* Planted and kept Cattle there; 5. of fuch Garden Herbs (amongft us) as do thrive there and of fuch as do not. 6. Of Stones, Minerals, Metals, and Earths.

Firft, Of Birds.[1]

The Humming Bird.

THe *Humming Bird*, the leaft of all Birds, little bigger than a *Dor*, of variable glittering Colours, they feed upon Honey, which they fuck out of Bloffoms [7] and Flowers with their long Needle-like Bills; they fleep all Winter, and are not to be feen till the Spring, at which time they breed in little Nefts, made up like a bottom of foft, Silk-like matter, their Eggs no bigger than a white Peafe, they hatch three or four at a time, and are proper to this Country.

---

[1] There is a much fuller account — to be noticed again — of our birds, in the Voyages. pp. 95-103. Wood's (N. E. Profpect, chap. viii.) is also curious. In the notes which immediately follow, on the birds, beasts, fishes, and reptiles, the oldest writers on our natural history will be found often to explain or illustrate each other.

The Troculus.[1]

The *Troculus*, a fmall Bird, black and white, no bigger than a Swallow, the points of whofe Feathers are fharp, which they ftick into the fides of the Chymney (to reft themfelves, their Legs being exceeding fhort) where they breed in Nefts made like a Swallows Neft, but of a glewy fubftance, and which is not faftened to the Chymney as a Swallows Neft, but hangs down the Chymney by a clew-like ftring a yard long. They commonly have four or five young ones, and when they go away, which is much about the time that Swallows ufe to depart, they never fail to throw down one of their young Birds into the room by way of Gratitude. I have more than once obferved, that againft the ruin of the Family thefe Birds will fuddenly forfake the houfe and come no more.

[8] The Pilhannaw.[2]

The *Pilhannaw* or *Mechquan*, much like the defcrip-tion of the *Indian Ruck*, a monftrous great Bird, a kind

---

[1] Chimney-swallow.

[2] "The pilhannaw is the king of birds of prey in New England. Some take him to be a kind of eagle; others for the Indian ruck, — the biggest bird that is, except the ostrich. One Mr. Hilton, living at Pascataway, had the hap to kill one of them. Being by the sea-side, he perceived a great shadow over his head, the sun shining out clear. Casting up his eyes, he saw a monstrous bird soaring aloft in the air; and, of a sudden, all the ducks and geese (there being then a great many) dived under water, nothing of them appearing but their heads. Mr. Hilton, having made readie his piece, shot and brought her down to the ground. How he disposed of her, I know not; but had he taken her alive, and sent her over into England, neither Bartholomew nor Sturbridge Fair could have produced such another sight." — *Josselyn's Voyages*, p. 95. These notices have been taken

of Hawk, fome fay an Eagle, four times as big as a Gof-hawk, white Mail'd, having two or three purple Feathers in her head as long as Geefes Feathers they make Pens of the Quills of thefe Feathers are purple, as big as Swans Quills and tranfparent; her Head is as big as a Childs of a year old, a very Princely Bird; when fhe foars abroad, all fort of feathered Creatures hide them-felves, yet fhe never preys upon any of them, but upon *Fawns* and *Jaccals:* She Ayries in the Woods upon the high Hills of *Offapy*, and is very rarely or feldome feen.

The Turkie.[1]

The *Turkie*, who is blacker than ours; I have heard feveral credible perfons affirm, they have feen *Turkie*

to be sufficient by some writers to show the probable existence of "a bird of prey, very large and bold, on the back of some of our American plantations." But our author's account indicates clearly a crested eagle, which we cannot explain by any thing nearer home than the yzquautli, or crested vulture of Mexico and the countries south of it (*Falco Harpyja*, Gmel.); two notices of which (cited by Linnæus) had been published some twenty years before Josselyn wrote, and may have been supposed by him to be applicable to a large bird which he had heard of as inhabiting mountains about Ossipee. The great heron — an inhabitant of the coast, and so uncommon inland that "one . . . shot in the upper parts of New Hampshire was described to" Wilson "as a great curiosity" (Amer. Ornith.. by Brewer. p. 555) — has the size and the crest of Josselyn's bird; and, if this last was only (as is possible) the name of a confused conception made up from several accounts of large birds, the heron may well be thought to have had a share in it.

[1] "Of these, sometimes there will be forty, threescore and a hundred, of a flock; sometimes more, and sometimes less. Their feeding is acorns, hawes, and berries: some of them get a haunt to frequent English corn. In winter, when the snow covers the ground, they resort to the seashore to look for shrimps, and such small fishes, at low tides. Such as love turkey-hunting must follow it in winter, after a new-fallen snow, when he may follow them by their tracks. Some have killed ten or a dozen in half a day. If they can be found towards an

Cocks that have weighed forty, yea fixty pound; but out
of my perfonal experimental knowledge I can affure you,
that I have eaten my fhare of a *Turkie Cock*, that when he
was pull'd and garbidg'd, weighed thirty [9] pound; and
I have alfo feen threefcore broods of young *Turkies* on
the fide of a marfh, sunning of themfelves in a morning
betimes, but this was thirty years fince, the *Englifh* and
the *Indians* having now deftroyed the breed, fo that 'tis
very rare to meet with a wild *Turkie* in the Woods; But
fome of the *Englifh* bring up great ftore of the wild kind,
which remain about their Houfes as tame as ours in
England.

The Goofe.[1]

The *Goofe*, of which there are three kinds; the *Gray
Goofe*, the *White Goofe*, and the *Brant:* The *Goofe* will

---

evening, and watched where they perch. — if one come about ten or eleven of the
clock, — he may shoot as often as he will : they will sit, unless they be slenderly
wounded. These turkies remain all the year long. The price of a good turkey-
cock is four shillings; and he is well worth it, for he may be in weight forty
pounds; a hen, two shillings."— *Wood, N. Eng. Prospect*, chap. viii. See also
Joffelyn's Voyages. p. 99.

[1] "The geese of the country be of three sorts. First. a brant goose; which is
a goose almost like the wild goose in England. The price of one of these is six-
pence. The second kind is a white goose, almost as big as an English tame
goose. These come in great flocks about Michaelmas : sometimes there will be
two or three thousand in a flock. Those continue six weeks, and so fly to the
southward; returning in March, and staying six weeks more, returning to
the northward. The price of one of these is eightpence. The third kind of
geese is a great grey goose, with a black neck, and a black and white head;
strong of flight : and these be a great deal bigger than the ordinary geese of
England; some very fat, and, in the spring, full of feathers, that the shot can
scarce pierce them. Most of these geese remain with us from Michaelmas to
April. They feed in the sea upon grass in the bays at low water, and gravel, and

live a long time; I once found in a *White Goose* three Hearts, fhe was a very old one, and fo tuff, that we gladly gave her over although exceeding well roafted.

The Bloody-Flux Cured.

A Friend of mine of good Quality living fometime in *Virginia* was fore troubled for a long time with the *Bloody-Flux*, having tryed feveral Remedies by the advice of his Friends without any good effect, at laft was induced with a longing defire to drink the *Fat Dripping* [10] of a Goofe newly taken from the Fire, which abfolutely cured him, who was in defpair of ever recovering his health again.

The Gripe and Vulture.

The *Gripe*, which is of two kinds, the one with a White Head, the other with a black Head, this we take for the *Vulture*. They are both cowardly *Kites*,[1] preying upon

---

in the woods of acorns; having, as other fowl have, their pass and repass to the northward and southward. The accurate marksmen kill of these both flying and sitting. The price of a grey goose is eighteen-pence."— *Wood, N. E. Prospect, l. c.* The white goose here mentioned is probably the snow-goose; upon which compare Nuttall. Mass. Ornith., Water-Birds, p. 344. Josselyn (Voyages, p. 100) says the brant and the gray goose "are best meat; the white are lean and tough, and live a long time; whereupon the proverb, 'Older than a white goose:'" which is not supported by Wood or later writers. The snow-goose has become much less frequent with us since the settlement of the country. The great grey goose of Wood is our well-known Canada goose.

[1] This was the best that our author could say of the eagles of New England. Wood assists us once more here : " The eagles of the country be of two sorts, — one like the eagles that be in England; the other is something bigger, with a great white head and white tail. These be commonly called gripes."— *New-Eng.*

Fifh caft up on the fhore. In the year 1668. there was a great mortality of Eels in *Cafco Bay*, thither reforted at the fame time an infinite number of *Gripes*, infomuch that being fhot by the Inhabitants, they fed their Hogs with them for fome weeks; at other times you fhall feldom fee above two or three in a dozen miles travelling. The *Quill Feathers* in their Wings make excellent *Text Pens*, and the Feathers of their Tail are highly efteemed by the *Indians* for their Arrows, they will not fing in flying; a *Gripes* Tail is worth a *Beavers* Skin, up in the Country.

Profpeā, l. c. The first spoken of by Wood — and perhaps, also, what Josselyn names last — may be the common or ring-tailed eagle, now known to be the young of the golden eagle. The second of Wood, and first of our author, is without doubt, the bald eagle; the (so to say) tyrannical habits of which bird are sufficiently well known, at least in the vivid pages of Wilson. See the Voyages, p. 96; where we learn also that "hawkes there are of several kinds; as goshawks, falcons, laniers, sparrow-hawkes, and a little black hawke highly prized by the Indians, who wear them on their heads, and is accounted of worth sufficient to ransom a sagamour. They are so strangely couragious and hardie that nothing flyeth in the air that they will not bind with. I have seen them tower so high, that they have been so small that scarcely could they be taken by the eye" (p. 95-6). Wood makes like mention of this little black hawk (New-Eng. Profpeā, l. c.); and R. Williams (Key into the Language of the Indians of N. E., in Hist. Coll., vol. iii. p. 220) calls it "sachim, a little bird about the bigness of a swallow, or less; to which the Indians give that name, because of its sachem or prince-like courage and command over greater birds: that a man shall often see this small bird pursue and vanquish and put to flight the crow and other birds far bigger than itself." This was our well-known king-bird; and Josselyn, on the same page, tells us of "a small ash-colour bird that is shaped like a hawke, with talons and beak, that falleth upon crowes; mounting up into the air after them, and will beat them till they make them cry:" which was, perhaps, the king-bird's half-cousin, as Wilson calls him, — the purple-martin.

A Remedy for the Coldnefs and pain of the Stomach.

The Skin of a *Gripe* dreft with the doun on, is good to wear upon the Stomach for the Pain and Coldnefs of it.

[11] *The Ofprey.*

The *Ofprey*, which in this Country is white mail'd.

A Remedy for the Tooth-ach.

Their Beaks excell for the Tooth-ach, picking the Gums therewith till they bleed.

The Wobble.[1]

The *Wobble*, an ill fhaped Fowl, having no long Feathers in their Pinions, which is the reafon they cannot fly, not much unlike the *Pengwin;* they are in the Spring very fat, or rather oyly, but pull'd and garbidg'd, and laid to the Fire to roaft, they yield not one drop.

For Aches.

Our way (for they are very foveraign for *Aches*) is to make Mummy of them, that is, to falt them well, and dry them in an earthern pot well glazed in an Oven; or elfe (which is the better way) to burn them under ground for a day or two, then quarter them and ftew them in a Tin Stewpan with a very little water.

---

[1] Nuttall (Manual, Water-Birds, p. 520) says that the young of the red-throated diver is called cobble in England. Our author elsewhere (Voyages, p. 101) makes mention of the "wobble" and the "wilmote" (that is, guillemot) as distinct; but *his* wilmot was "a kind of teal."

[12] *The Loone.*

The *Loone* is a Water Fowl, alike in fhape to the *Wobble*, and as virtual for Aches, which we order after the fame manner.[1]

The Owl.

The *Owl, Avis devia,* which are of three kinds; the great *Gray Owl* with Ears, the little *Gray Owl,* and the *White Owl* which is no bigger than a *Thrufh.*[2]

The Turkie Buzzard.

The *Turkie Buzzard,* a kind of *Kite,* but as big as a *Turkie,* brown of colour, and very good meat.[3]

What Birds are not to be found in New-England.

Now, by what the country hath not, you may ghefs at what it hath; it hath no *Nightingals,* nor *Larks,* nor *Bulfinches,* nor *Sparrows,* nor *Blackbirds,* nor *Mag*[12]*pies,*

---

[1] "He maketh a noise sometimes like a sow-gelder's horn." — *N. Eng. Profpeꝗ, l. c.*

[2] The first is the great-horned or cat-owl; the second, probably, the mottled or little screech-owl, which Wood notices more fully as "small, speckled like a partridge, with ears" (*l. c.*); and the third, the Acadian or little owl. There are but two owls reckoned in New-England's Profpect; the second of which — "a great owl, almost as big as an eagle; his body being as good meat as a partridge" (*l. c.*) — is, perhaps, the snowy owl, which, according to Audubon, is good eating. — *Peabody Report on Birds of Mass.,* p. 275.

[3] It is not clear what is meant here. The author merely mentions the bird again, in Voyages, p. 96.

nor *Jackdawes*, nor *Popinjays*, nor *Rooks*, nor *Pheasants*, nor *Woodcocks*, nor *Quails*, nor *Robins*, nor *Cuckoes*, &c.[1]

---

[1] So Wood: "There are no magpies, jackdaws, cuckoos, jays, &c." — *New-England's Prospect, l. c.* Our author, in his Voyages, adds to the above list of New-England birds the following: "The partridge is larger than ours; white-flesht, but very dry: they are indeed a sort of partridges called grooses. The pidgeon, of which there are millions of millions. . . . The snow-bird, like a chaffinch, go in flocks, and are good meat. . . . Thrushes, with red breasts, which will be very fat, and are good meat. . . . Thressels, . . . filladies, . . . small singing-birds; ninmurders, little yellow birds; New-England nightingales, painted with orient colours, — black, white, blew, yellow, green, and scarlet, — and sing sweetly; wood-larks, wrens, swallows, who will sit upon trees; and starlings, black as ravens, with scarlet pinions. Other sorts of birds there are; as the troculus, wagtail or dish-water, which is here of a brown colour; titmouse, — two or three sorts; the dunneck or hedge-sparrow, who is starke naked in his winter nest; the golden or yellow hammer, — a bird about the bigness of a thrush, that is all over as red as bloud; woodpeckers of two or three sorts, gloriously set out with variety of glittering colours; the colibry, viemalin, or rising or walking-bird, — an emblem of the resurrection, and the wonder of little birds. The water-fowl are these that follow: Hookers, or wild swans; cranes; . . . four sorts of ducks, — a black duck, a brown duck like our wild ducks, a grey duck, and a great black and white duck. These frequent rivers and ponds. But, of ducks, there be many more sorts: as hounds, old wives, murres, doies, shell-drakes, shoulers or shoflers, widgeons, simps, teal, blew-wing'd and green-wing'd didapers or dipchicks, fenduck, duckers or moorhens, coots, pochards (a water-fowl like a duck), plungeons (a kind of water-fowl, with a long, reddish bill), puets, plovers, smethes, wilmotes (a kind of teal), godwits, humilities, knotes, red-shankes, . . . gulls, white gulls or sea-cobbs, caudemandies, herons, grey bitterns, ox-eyes, birds called oxen and keen, petterels, king's fishers, . . . little birds that frequent the sea-shore in flocks, called sanderlins. They are about the bigness of a sparrow, and, in the fall of the leaf, will be all fat. When I was first in the countrie " (that is, in 1638; in which connection, what follows is not without its interest to us), " the English cut them into small pieces to put into their puddings, instead of suet. I have known twelve-score and above killed at two shots. . . . The cormorant, shape or sharke " (pp. 99-103).

Secondly, Of Beafts.[1]

The Bear, which are generally Black.[2]

THe *Bear*, they live four months in Caves, that is all Winter; in the Spring they bring forth their young ones, they feldome have above three Cubbs in a litter, are very fat in the Fall of the Leaf with feeding upon Acorns, at which time they are excellent Venifon; their Brains are venomous; They feed much upon water Plantane in the Spring and Summer, and Berries, and alfo upon a fhell-fifh called a *Horfe-foot;* and are never mankind, i.e. fierce, but in rutting time, and then they walk the Country twenty, thirty, forty in a company, making a hideous noife with roaring, which you may hear a mile or two before they come fo near to endanger the Traveller. About four years fince, Acorns being very fcarce up in the Country, fome numbers of them came down [14] amongft the *English* Plantations, which generally are by the Sea fide;

---

[1] Compare the account given in the Voyages, pp. 82–95, which is much fuller; as also New-England's Prospect, chap. vi.

[2] "Most fierce in strawberry-time; at which time they have young ones; at which time, likewise, they will go upright, like a man, and climb trees, and swim to the islands: which if the Indians see, there will be more sportful bear-baiting than Paris garden can afford; for, seeing the bears take water, an Indian will leap after him; where they go to water-cuffs for bloody noses and scratched sides. In the end. the man gets the victory; riding the bear over the watery plain, till he can bear him no longer. . . . There would be more of them, if it were not for the wolves which devour them. A kennel of those ravening runagadoes, setting upon a poor, single bear, will tear him as a dog will tear a kid." — *New-Eng. Prospect, l. c.,* which see farther; and also Josselyn's Voyages, pp. 91-2.

at one Town called *Gorgiana* in the Province of *Meyn* (called alfo *New-Sommerfet-fhire*) they kill'd fourfcore.

For Aches and Cold Swellings.

Their Greafe is very good for Aches and Cold Swellings, the *Indians* anoint themfelves therewith from top to toe, which hardens them againft the cold weather. A black Bears Skin heretofore was worth forty fhillings, now you may have one for ten, much ufed by the *Englifh* for Beds and Coverlets, and by the *Indians* for Coats.

For Pain and Lamenefs upon Cold.

One *Edw. Andrews* being foxt,[1] and falling backward crofs a Thought[2] in a Shallop or Fifher-boat, and taking cold upon it, grew crooked, lame, and full of pain, was cured, lying one Winter upon Bears Skins newly flead off, with fome upon him, fo that he fweat every night.

The Wolf.[3]

The *Wolf*, of which there are two kinds; one with a round-ball'd Foot, and [15] are in fhape like mungrel

---

[1] Stupefied with drink. — *Webster, Eng. Dict.*

[2] Thwart.

[3] "The woolves be in some respect different from them in other countries. It was never known yet that a wolf ever set upon a man or woman: neither do they trouble horses or cows; but swine, goats, and red calves, which they take for deer. be often destroyed by them; so that a red calf is cheaper than a black one, in that regard. in some places. . . . They be made much like a mungrel; being big-boned, lank-paunched, deep-breasted; having a thick neck and head, prick ears and long snout, with dangerous teeth; long, staring hair, and a great bush-tail. It is thought by many that our English mastiff might be too hard for them:

Maftiffs; the other with a flat Foot, thefe are liker Grey-
hounds, and are called *Deer Wolfs*, because they are
accuftomed to prey upon *Deer*.　A *Wolf* will eat a *Wolf*
new dead, and fo do *Bears* as I fuppofe, for their dead
Carkafes are never found, neither by the *Indian* nor
Englifh.　They go a clicketing twelve days, and have as
many Whelps at a Litter as a Bitch.　The *Indian Dog*[1] is
a Creature begotten 'twixt a *Wolf* and a *Fox*, which the
Indians lighting upon, bring up to hunt the *Deer* with.
The *Wolf* is very numerous, and go in companies, fometimes ten, twenty, more or fewer, and fo cunning, that
feldome any are kill'd with Guns or Traps; but of late
they have invented a way to deftroy them, by binding four
Maycril Hooks a crofs with a brown thread, and then
wrapping fome Wool about them, they dip them in melted
Tallow till it be as round and as big as an Egg; thefe
(when any Beaft hath been kill'd by the *Wolves*) they
fcatter by the dead Carkafe, after they have beaten off the
Wolves; about Midnight the *Wolves* are fure to return
again to the place where they left the flaughtered Beaft,
and the (16) firft thing they venture upon will be thefe
balls of fat.

---

but it is no such matter: for they care no more for an ordinary mastiff than an
ordinary mastiff cares for a cur.　Many good dogs have been spoiled by
them. . . . There is little hope of their utter destruction; the country being so
spacious, and they so numerous, travelling in the swamps by kennels: sometimes
ten or twelve are of a company. . . . In a word, they be the greatest inconven-
iency the country hath." — *New-England's Profpect, l. c.*

[1] Spoken of again in the Voyages, pp. 94 and 193; and in Hubbard, Hist.
N. England, p. 25.　Josselyn's may be compared with Lewis and Clark's notice of
the Indian dog (Travels, vol. ii. p. 165).

For old Aches.

A black *Wolfs* Skin is worth a *Beaver* Skin among the *Indians*, being highly efteemed for helping old Aches in old people, worn as a Coat; they are not mankind, as in *Ireland* and other Countries, but do much harm by deftroying of our *Englifh* Cattle.

The Ounce.[1]

The *Ounce* or *Wild Cat*, is about the bignefs of two lufty Ram Cats, preys upon Deer and our *Englifh* Poultrey: I once found fix whole Ducks in the belly of one I killed by a Pond fide: Their flefh roafted is as good as Lamb, and as white.

For Aches and fhrunk Sinews.

Their Greafe is foveraign for all manner of Aches and fhrunk Sinews: Their Skins are accounted good Fur, but fomewhat courfe.

---

[1] Called also "lusern, or luceret," in the Voyages, p. 85; the loup-cervier of Sagard (Hist. Can., 1636, *cit.* Aud. and Bachm. Vivip. Quad. N. A., p. 136); of Dobbs's Hudson's Bay, &c.; but more commonly called gray cat, or lynx, in New.England. Wood calls it "more dangerous to be met withal than any other creature; not fearing either dog or man. He useth to kill deer. . . . He hath likewise a device to get geese: for, being much of the colour of a goose, he will place himself close by the water; holding up his bob-tail, which is like a goose-neck. The geese. seeing this counterfeit goose, approach nigh to visit him; who, with a sudden jerk, apprehends his mistrustless prey. The English kill many of these. accounting them very good meat." — *New-Eng.'Prospect, l. c.* Audubon and Bachman (*l. c.*, p. 14) give a similar good account of the flesh of the bay-lynx. or common wild-cat.

[17] *The Raccoon.*[1]

The *Raccoon* liveth in hollow trees, and is about the fize of a *Gib Cat;* they feed upon Mafs, and do infeft our *Indian* Corn very much; they will be exceeding fat in Autumn; their flefh is fomewhat dark, but good food roafted.

For Bruifes and Aches.

Their Fat is excellent for bruifes and Aches. Their Skins are efteemed a good deep Fur; but yet as the *Wild Cats* fomewhat coarfe.

The Porcupine.

The *Porcupine*, in fome parts of the Countrey Eaftward towards the *French*, are as big as an ordinary Mungrel Cur; a very angry Creature, and dangerous, fhooting a whole fhower of Quills with a rowfe at their enemies, which are of that nature, that wherever they ftick in the flefh, they will work through in a fhort time, if not prevented by pulling of them out. The *Indians* make ufe of their Quills, which are hardly a handful long, to adorn [18] the edges of their birchen difhes, and weave (dying

---

[1] The raccoon is, or has been, an inhabitant of all North America (Godman, Nat. Hist., vol. i. p. 117), and was one of the firft of our animals with which European naturalists became acquainted. Linnæus (Syft. Nat.) cites Conrad Gefner among thofe who have illustrated or mentioned it. Wood fays they are "as good meat as a lamb;" and further, that, "in the moonshine night, they go to feed on clams at a low tide, by the seaside, where the English hunt them with their dogs." — *New-Eng. Profpect, l. c.*

fome of them red, others yellow and blew) curious bags
or pouches, in works like *Turkic-work.*[1]

The Beaver, Canis Ponticus, Amphybious.[2]

The *Beaver,* whofe old ones are as big as an *Otter,* or
rather bigger, a Creature of a rare inftinct, as may apparently be feen in their artificial Dam-heads to raife the
water in the Ponds where they keep, and their houfes
having three ftories, which would be too large to dif-
courfe.[2] They have all of them four Cods hanging out-
wardly between their hinder legs, two of them are foft or
oyly, and two folid or hard; the *Indians* fay they are
Hermaphrodites.

For Wind in the Stomach.

• Their folid Cods are much ufed in Phyfick: Our *Englifh-
women* in this Country ufe the powder grated, as much as
will lye upon a fhilling in a draught of *Fiol* Wine, for
Wind in the Stomach and Belly, and venture many times
in fuch cafes to give it to Women with Child: Their
Tails are flat, and covered with Scales without hair, [19]
which being flead off, and the Tail boiled, proves exceeding good meat, being all Fat, and as fweet as Marrow.

---

[1] The author's account of the Indian works in birch-bark and porcupine-quills
is much fuller in his Voyages, p. 143.
[2] Wood's account is far better. — *New-Eng. Prospect,* chap. vii. See page 53
of the Rarities for mention of the musk quash.

The Moofe-Deer.[1]

The *Moofe Deer*, which is a very goodly Creature, fome of them twelve foot high, with exceeding fair Horns with broad Palms, fome of them two fathom from the tip of one Horn to the other; they commonly have three *Fawns* at a time, their flefh is not dry like Deers flefh, but moift and lufhious fomewhat like Horfe flefh (as they judge that have tafted of both) but very wholfome. The flefh of their *Fawns* is an incomparable difh, beyond the flefh of an Affes Foal fo highly efteemed by the *Romans*, or that of young Spaniel Puppies fo much cried up in our days in *France* and *England*.

Moofe Horns better for Phyfick Ufe than Harts Horns.

Their Horns are far better (in my opinion) for Phyfick than the Horns of other Deer, as being of a ftronger nature: As for their Claws, which both *Englifhmen* and *French* make ufe of for *Elk*, I cannot [20] approve fo to be from the Effects, having had fome trial of it; befides,

---

[1] See Voyages, pp. 88-91. Called *moos-soog* (rendered "great-ox; or, rather, red deer") in R. Williams's Key (Hist. Coll., vol. iii. p. 223): but this is rather the plural form of *moos*; as fee the fame, *l. c.* p. 222, and note, and Rasles' Dict. Abnaki, *in loco*. It is called *mongfüa* by the Cree Indians; and, it should seem, *mongsoos* by the Indians of the neighborhood of Carlton House; as see Richardson, in Sabine's Appendix to Franklin's Narrative of a Journey to the Polar Sea, pp. 665-6. "The English," says Wood, "have fome thoughts of keeping him tame, and to accustome him to the yoke; which will be a great commodity. . . . There be not many of these in the Massachusetts Bay; but, forty miles to the north-east, there be great store of them." — *New-Eng. Prospect, l. c.* On hunting the moose, as practised by the Indians, see Josselyn's Voyages, p. 136.

all that write of the *Elk* defcribe him with a tuft of hair
on the left Leg behind, a little above the paftern joynt on
the outfide of the Leg, not unlike the tuft (as I conceive)
that groweth upon the breaft of a *Turkie Cock*, which I
could never yet fee upon the Leg of a *Moofe*, and I have
feen fome number of them.

For Children breeding Teeth.

The *Indian Webbes* make ufe of the broad Teeth of the
Fawns to hang about their Childrens Neck when they are
breeding of their Teeth. The Tongue of a grown *Moofe*,
dried in the fmoak after the *Indian* manner, is a difh for a
Sagamor.

The Maccarib.[1]

The *Maccarib*, *Caribo*, or *Pohano*, a kind of Deer, as
big as a Stag, round hooved, fmooth hair'd and foft as filk;

---

[1] Wood (N. E. Prospect, *l. c.*) has but two kinds of deer: of which the first is
the moose; and the second, called "ordinary deer," and, in the vocabulary of
Indian words, *ottuck* (compare *attuck* or *noonatch*, deer, — R. Williams, *l. c.;* ⃰
but *atteyk*, in the Cree dialect, signifies a small sort of rein-deer, — Richardson,
in Appendix to Franklin's Journey, p. 665; and it is observable that Rasles' word
for *chevreuil* is *norke*), is our American fallow-deer. R. Williams also appears
to distinguish with clearness but two; which are, perhaps, the same as Wood's.
Josselyn, in this book, passes quite over the common, or fallow-deer: but, making
up in the Voyages for the fallings-short of the Rarities, he goes, in the former,
quite the other way; reckoning the roe, buck, red deer, rein-deer, elk, *maurouse*,
and *maccarib*. What is further said of these animals, where he speaks more at
large, makes it appear likely that the second, third, and fourth names, so far as
they have any value, belong to a single kind, — the "ordinary deer" of Wood
(whose description possibly helped Josselyn's), or our fallow-deer; to which the
"roe" is also to be referred: and the "elk" he himself explains as the moose.
But, beside these two kinds, Josselyn has the merit of indicating, with some

their Horns grow backwards a long their backs to their rumps, and turn again a handful beyond their Nofe, having another Horn in the middle of their Forehead, about half a yard long, very ftraight, but [21] wreathed like an *Unicorns* Horn, of a brown jettie colour, and very fmooth: The Creature is no where to be found, but upon Cape *Sable* in the *French* Quarters, and there too very rarely, they being not numerous; fome few of their Skins and their ftreight Horns are (but very fparingly) brought to the *Englifh*.

The Fox.[1]

The *Fox*, which differeth not much from ours, but are fomewhat lefs; a black *Fox* Skin heretofore was wont to

---

distinctness, one, or possibly two, others, — the *maurouse* and the *maccarib*. The *maurouse* — of which only the Voyages make mention — "is somewhat like a moose; but his horns are but small, and himself about the size of a stag. These are the deer that the flat-footed wolves hunt after." — *Voyages*, p. 91. This is to be compared with the *mauroos*, rendered "*cerf*," of Rasles' Dict., *l. c.*, p. 382; and, in such connection, is hardly referable to other than the *caribou*, or reindeer, — a well-known inhabitant of the north-eastern parts of New England, and likely, therefore, to have come to the knowledge of our author; while there seems to be no testimony to its ever having occurred in Massachusetts and southward, where Wood and Williams made their observations. The last, or the *maccarib*, *caribo*, or *pohano*, of Josselyn, is described above; and, in the Voyages (p. 91), he only repeats that it "is not found, that ever I heard yet, but upon Cape Sable, near to the French plantations." The "round" hoofs of the *maccarib* might lead us to take this for the *caribou* of Maine; the round track of which differs much from that of the fallow-deer. But the former is more likely to have been the American elk; so rare, it should seem, where it occurred, when our author wrote, and so little known in the New-England settlements, that his fancy, fed by darkling hearsay, could deck it with the honors of the "unicorn."

[1] "There are two or three kinds of them, — one a great yellow fox; another grey, who will climb up into trees. The black fox is of much esteem." — *Josse-*

be valued at fifty and fixty pound, but now you may have them for twenty fhillings; indeed there is not any in *New-England* that are perfectly black, but filver hair'd, that is fprinkled with grey hairs.

The Jaccal.[1]

The *Jaccal*, is a Creature that hunts the *Lions* prey, a fhrew'd fign that there are *Lions* upon the Continent; there are thofe that are yet living in the Countrey, that do conftantly affirm, that about fix or feven and thirty years fince an *Indian* [22] fhot a young *Lion*,[2] fleeping upon the body

---

lyn's Voyages, p. 82; where is also an account of the way of hunting foxes in New England. Wood has nothing special, but that some of the foxes " be black. Their furrs is of much esteem " (*l. c.*) Williams (*l. c.*) has " *mishquashim*, a red fox; *pequawus*, a gray fox. The Indians say they have black foxes, which they have often seen, but never could take any of them. They say they are manittooes." Beside the common red fox, or *mishquashim*, we have in all these accounts — and also in Morell's *Nova Anglia, l. c.*, p. 129 — mention of a black fox; which may have been the true black or silver fox, or, in part at least, the more common cross-fox (Aud. and Bachm., Viv. Quadr. N. A., p. 45); the pelt of which is also in high esteem. For Williams's gray fox, see the next note. Josselyn's climbing gray fox is perhaps the fisher (*Mustela Canadensis*, Schreb.), notwithstanding the color. According to Audubon (*l. c.*, pp. 51, 310, 315), this is called the black fox in New England and the northern counties of New York. I have heard it more often called black cat in New Hampshire. But the true gray fox (*Vulpes Virginianus*) " has, to a certain degree, the power of climbing trees." Newberry Zoology, Expl. for Pacific Railroad, vi, part 4, p. 40.

1 "A creature much like a fox, but smaller." — *Voyages*, p. 83. Probably the gray fox, called *pequawus* by R. Williams (*Vulpes Virginianus*, Schreb.); which has not the rank smell of the red fox. — *Aud. and Bachm., l. c.*, p. 168.

2 " They told me of a young lyon (not long before) kill'd at Piscataway by an Indian." — *Voyages*, p. 23. Higginson says that lions " have been seen at Cape Anne." — *New-Eng. Plantation, l. c.*, p. 119. " Some affirm," says Wood, " that they have seen a lion at Cape Anne. . . . Besides, Plimouth men" (that is, men of old Plymouth, it is likely) " have traded for lion-skins in former times. But

H

of an Oak blown up by the roots, with an Arrow, not far from Cape *Anne*, and fold the Skin to the *Englifh*. But to fay fomething of the *Jaccal*, they are ordinarily lefs than *Foxes*, of the colour of a gray Rabbet, and do not fcent nothing near fo ftrong as a *Fox;* some of the *Indians* will eat of them: Their Greafe is good for all that *Fox* Greafe is good for, but weaker; they are very numerous.

The Hare.[1]

The *Hare* in *New-England* is no bigger than our *Englifh* Rabbets, of the fame colour, but withall having yellow and black ftrokes down the ribs; in Winter they are milk white, and as the Spring approacheth they come to their colour; when the Snow lies upon the ground they are very bitter with feeding upon the bark of Spruce, and the like.[2]

---

sure it is that there be lions on that continent; for the Virginians saw an old lion in their plantation," &c. — *New-Eng. Prospect, l. c.* The animal here spoken of may well have been the puma or cougar, or American lion.

[1] "The rabbits be much like ours in England. The hares be some of them white, and a yard long. These two harmless creatures are glad to shelter themselves from the harmful foxes in hollow trees; having a hole at the entrance no bigger than they can creep in at." — *Wood, New-Eng. Prospect, l. c.* Wood's rabbit and Josselyn's hare, so far as the summer coloring goes, appear to be the gray rabbit (*Lepus sylvaticus*, Aud. and Bachm., *l. c.* p. 173); and the white hare of Wood — as also, probably, the hare, "milk-white in winter," of Josselyn — is doubtless the northern hare (*Lepus Americanus*, Erxl., Aud. and Bachm., *l. c.*, p. 93).

[2] The Voyages mention, beside the quadrupeds above named, also the skunk (*ségañkoo* of Rasles' Dict., *l. c.*); the musquash (*mooskooéssoo* of Rasles, *l. c.*), for

[23] Thirdly, Of Fiſhes.[1]

P*Liny* and *Iſadore* write there are not above 144 Kinds of Fiſhes, but to my knowledge there are nearer 300: I ſuppoſe *America* was not known to *Pliny* and *Iſadore*.

---

which see also p. 53 of this; otter; marten, "as ours are in England, but blacker;" sable, "much of the size of a mattrise, perfect black, but . . . I never saw but two of them in eight years' space;" the squirrel, "three sorts, — the mouse-squirril, the gray squirril, and the flying-squirril (called by the Indian *assapanick*)." Our author's mouse-squirrel, which he describes, is the ground or striped squirrel: probably the "*anequus*, a little coloured squirrel" of R. Williams, *l. c.*; and the *anikoosess* (rendered *suisse*) of Rasles, *l. c.* The mattrise of our author is, according to him, "a creature whose head and fore-parts is shaped somewhat like a lyon's; not altogether so big as a house-cat. They are innumerable up in the countrey, and are esteemed good furr." — *Voyages*, p. 87. The sable is compared with the mattrise, at least in size; and the name is perhaps comparable with *mattegooéssoo* of Rasles, *l. c.*; but this is rendered *lièvre*. Wood adds to this list of our quadrupeds, mistakenly, the ferret; and R. Williams, the "*ockquutchaun-nug*, — a wild beast of a reddish hair, about the bigness of a pig, and rooting like a pig;" which seems to answer, in name as well as habits, to our woodchuck, or ground-hog.

1 The author's attempt here at a general catalogue of the fishes, mollusks, &c., of the North-Atlantic Ocean, affords but a poor make-shift for such a list as we might fairly have expected from him of the species known to the early fishermen in the waters and seas of New England; and the account in his Voyages (pp. 104-15) is again an improvement on the present, and is confined to the inhabitants of our waters. The present editor has little to offer in elucidation of the list; which indeed, in good part, appears sufficiently intelligible. Compare Wood, New-Eng. Prospect, chap. x.

A Catalogue of Fiſh, that is, of thoſe that are to be ſeen between the Engliſh Coaſt and America, *and thoſe proper to the Countrey.*

Alderling.

Alize, Alewife, becauſe great-bellied ; *Olaſe, Oldwife, Allow.*[1]

Anchova or *Sea Minnow.*

Aleport.

Albicore.[2]

Barble.

Barracha.

Barracoutha, a fiſh peculiar to the *Weſt-Indies.*[3]

Barſticle.

Baſſe.[4]

---

[1] "Like a herrin, but has a bigger bellie; therefore called an alewife." — *Voyages,* p. 107. The other names, alize and allow, are doubtless corruptions of the French *aloſe,* also in use among London fiſhmongers to designate shad from certain waters. — *Rees's Cyc., in loco.* The old Latin word *alosa,* supposed to have been always applied to the fish just mentioned, is adopted by Cuvier for the genus which includes our shad, alewife, and menhaden.

[2] The tunny is so called on the coast of New England. — *Storer's Report on the Fishes of Mass.,* p. 48.

[3] It is, notwithstanding, set down in the author's list of fishes "that are to be seen and catch'd in the sea and fresh waters in New England." — *Voyages,* p. 113. And compare Storer, Synops. (Mem. Am. Acad., N. S., vol. ii.), p. 300.

[4] See Voyages, p. 108. The first settlers esteemed the bass above most other fish. See Higginson's New-England's Plantation (Hist. Coll., vol. i. p. 120). Wood calls it (New-Eng. Prospect, chap. ix.) "one of the best fish in the country; and though men are soon wearied with other fish, yet are they never with bass. The Indians," he says, eat lobsters, "when they can get no bass." The head was especially prized; as see Wood, and also Roger Williams's Key (Hist. Coll., vol.

Sea Bishop, proper to the *Norway* Seas.

[24] *River Bleak* or *Bley*, a *River Swallow*.

Sea Bleak or *Bley*, or *Sea Camelion*.

Blew Fish or *Hound Fish*, two kinds, *speckled Hound Fish*, and *Blew Hound Fish* called *Horse Fish*.[1]

Bonito or *Dozado*, or *Spanish Dolphin*.[2]

River Bream.

Sea Bream.[3]

Cud Bream.

Bullhead or *Indian Muscle.*

River Bulls.

Burfish.

Burret.

Cackarel or *Laxe.*

Calemarie or *Sea Clerk.*

Catfish.[4]

Carp.

Chare, a *Fish* proper to the River *Wimander* in *Lancashire.*

Sea Chough.

Chub or *Chevin.*

Cony Fish.

---

iii. p. 224). The fish is our striped bass (*Labrax lineatus*, Cuv.; Storer's Report on Fishes of Mass., p. 7). Our author, at p. 37, again mentions it as one of the eight fishes which "the Indians have in greatest request."

[1] See p. 96 as to the blue-fish, or horse-mackerel; and Storer, *l. c.*, p. 57.

[2] The bonito of our fishermen is the skipjack. — *Storer, l. c.*, p. 49.

[3] See p. 95.

[4] See p. 96. Josselyn's character of the fish as food is confirmed by Dr. Storer, *l. c.*, p. 69.

Clam or *Clamp.*[1]
Sea Cob.
Cockes, or *Coccles,* or *Coquil.*[2]
Cook Fiſh.
Rock Cod.
Sea Cod or *Sea Whiting.*[3]
[25] *Crab,* divers kinds, as the *Sea Crab, Boatfiſh, River
Crab, Sea Lion, &c.*

---

[1] The clam is one of the eight fishes mentioned at p. 37 as most prized by the
Indians. "*Sickishuog* (clams). This is a sweet kind of shell-fish, which all
Indians generally over the country, winter and summer, delight in; and, at low
water, the women dig for them. This fish, and the natural liquor of it, they boil;
and it makes their broth and their nasaump (which is a kind of thickened broth)
and their bread seasonable and savoury, instead of salt." — *Williams's Key, &c.,
l. c.* p. 224. "These fishes be in great plenty in most parts of the country: which
is a great commodity for the feeding of swine, both in winter and summer; for,
being once used to those places, they will repair to them as duly, every ebb, as if
they were driven to them by keepers." — *Wood, N. Eng. Prospect, l. c.* The
mollusk thus approved is the common clam (*Mya arenaria,* L.); but the *poquau-
hock,* or quahog (*Venus mercenaria,* L.), "which the Indians wade deep and dive
for" (R. Williams, *l. c.,* p. 224), was also eaten by them, and the black part of
the shell used for making their *suckauhock,* or black money. Wood speaks also
of "clams as big as a penny white loaf, which are great dainties amongst the
natives" (N. E. Prospect, *l. c.*); doubtless the giant clam (*Mactra solidissima,*
Chemn.) of Gould (Report on Invertebr. of Mass., p. 51), which is still esteemed
as food.

[2] See p. 36; by which it appears that the author has in view the *metcauhock*
of the Indians; "the periwinkle, of which they make their *wompam,* or white
money, of half the value of their *suckauhock,* or black money" (R. Williams, *l. c.*):
supposed to be *Buccinum undatum,* L. (Gould, *l. c.,* p. 305); and possibly, also,
one or two other allied shell-fish.

[3] "Cod-fish in these seas" (that is, Massachusetts Bay) "are larger than in
Newfoundland, — six or seven making a quintal; whereas they have fifteen to
the same weight." — *New-Eng. Prospect, l. c.* Compare Storer, *l. c.,* p. 121.
Josselyn has an entertaining account of the sea-fishery, in his Voyages, pp.
210–13.

Sea Cucumber.

Cunger or *Sea Eel.*

Cunner or *Sea Roach.*

Cur.

Currier, Poſt, or *Lacquey* of the Sea.

Crampfiſh or *Torpedo.*

Cuttle, or *Sleeves,* or *Sea Angler.*

Clupea, the *Tunnies* enemy.

Sea Cornet.

Cornuta or *Horned Fiſh.*

Dace, Dare, or *Dart.*

Sea Dart, Javelins.

Dog-fiſh or *Tubarone.*

Dolphin.

Dorce.

Dorrie, Goldfiſh.

Golden-eye, Gilt-pole, or *Godline, Yellow-heads.*

Sea Dragon or *Sea Spider, Quaviner.*

Drum, a Fiſh frequent in the *Weſt Indies.*

Sea Emperour or *Sword Fiſh.*

Eel, of which divers kinds.[1]

Sea Elephant, the Leather of this Fiſh will never rot, excellent for Thongs.

Ears of the Sea.

---

[1] See further of eels, and the author's several ways of cooking them, in his Voyages, p. III. At p. 37 of the Rarities, eels are mentioned among the fishes most prized by the Indians. "These eels be not of so luscious a taste as they be in England, neither are they so aguish; but are both wholesome for the body, and delightful for the taste."— *Wood, New-Eng. Prospect,* chap. ix.

Flayl-fish.

[26] *Flownder* or *Flook*, the young ones are called *Dabs.*

Sea Flownder or *Flowre.*

Sea Fox.

Frogfish.

Frostfish.[1]

Frutola, a broad plain Fish with a Tail like a half Moon.

Sea Flea.

Gallyfish.

Grandpiss[2] or *Herring Hog*, this, as all Fish of extraordinary fize, are accounted Regal Fishes.

Grayling.

Greedigut.

Groundling.

Gudgin.

Gulf.

Sea Grape.

Gull.

Gurnard.

Hake.

Haccle or *Sticklebacks.*

Haddock.

Horfe Foot or *Affes Hoof.*

Herring.

---

[1] See p. 37, where it is said to be one of the fishes which "the Indians have in greatest request." — "*Poponaumsuog*" of R. Williams, *l. c.,* p. 225. He says, "Some call them frost-fish, from their coming up from the sea into fresh brooks in times of frost and snow."

[2] "Grampoise; Fr. *grandpoisson;*" corrupted grampus. — *Webster, Dict.*

Hallibut or *Sea Pheafant.* Some will have the *Turbut* all one, others diftinguifh [27] them, calling the young Fifh of the firft *Buttis,* and of the other *Birt.* There is no queftion to be made of it but that they are diftinct kinds of Fifh.[1]

Sea Hare.[2]

Sea Hawk.

Hartfifh.

Sea Hermit.

Henfifh.

Sea Hind.

Hornbeak, Sea Ruff and *Reeves.*

Sea Horfeman.

Hog or *Flying Fifh.*

Sea Kite or *Flying Swallow.*

Lampret or *Lamprel.*

Lampreys or *Lamprones.*[3]

Limpin.

Ling, Sea Beef; the fmaller fort is called *Cusk.*

Sea Lanthorn.

Sea Liver.

---

[1] "These hollibut be little set by while bass is in season." — *Wood, l. c.,* chap. ix.

[2] "The sea-hare is as big as grampus, or herrin-hog; and as white as a sheet. There hath been of them in Black-Point Harbour, and some way up the river; but we could never take any of them. Several have shot sluggs at them, but lost their labour." — *Voyages,* p. 105. The *Lepus marinus* of the old writers is a naked mollusk of the Mediterranean; *Laplysia depilans,* L.: but Josselyn's was a very different animal.

[3] One of the fishes most valued by the Indians (p. 37); but "not much set by" by the English, according to Wood, *l. c.*

I

Lobſter.[1]
Sea Lizard.
Sea Locuſts.
Lump, Poddle, or *Sea Owl.*
Lauter.
Lux, peculiar to the river *Rhyne.*
Sea Lights.

[28] *Luna,* a very ſmall Fiſh, but exceeding beautiful, broad-bodied and blewiſh of colour; when it ſwims, the Fins make a Circle like the Moon.

Maycril.
Maid.
Manatee.
Mola, a Fiſh like a lump of Fleſh, taken in the *Venetian* Sea.
Millers Thumb, Mulcet or *Pollard.*
Molefiſh.
Minnow, called likewiſe a *Pink;* the ſame name is given to young *Salmon;* it is called alſo a *Witlin.*
Monkcfiſh.[2]

---

[1] "I have seene some myselfe that have weighed 16 pound; but others have had, divers times, so great lobsters as have weighed 25 pound, as they assure me." — *Higginson's New-Eng. Plantation, l. c.,* p. 120; with which compare Gould's Report, &c., p. 360. "Their plenty makes them little esteemed, and seldom eaten." — *Wood, New-Eng. Prospect.* chap. ix. At p. 37, Josselyn counts them among the fishes, &c., most esteemed by the Indians; but Wood (*l. c.*) qualifies this in a passage already cited. The Indians, it seems, sometimes dried them, "as they do lampres and oysters; which are delicate breakfast-meat so ordered." — *Josselyn's Voyages,* p. 110. See the Indian way of catching lobsters, in Voyages, p. 140.

[2] "Munk-fish, a flat-fish like scate; having a hood like a fryer's cowl" (p. 96)· *Lophius Americanus,* Cuv., the sea-devil of Storer (Synops. of Amer. Fishes, in

Morfe, River or *Sea Horfe*,[1] frefh water *Mullet*.
Sea Mullet. Botargo or *Petargo* is made of their Spawn.
Mufcle, divers kinds.[2]
Navelfifh.
Nunfifh.
Needlefifh.
Sea Nettle.
Oyfter.[3]
Occulata.
Perch or *River Partridge*.
Pollack.
[29] *Piper* or *Gavefifh*.
Periwig.
Periwincle or *Sea Snail* or *Whelk*.
Pike, or *Frefh-water Wolf*, or *River Wolf*, *Luce* and
Lucerne, which is an overgrown *Pike*.
Pilchard, when they are dried as *Red Herrings* they are
called *Fumadoes*.
Pilot Fifh.
Plaice or *Sea Sparrow*.
Polipe or *Pour-Contrel*.

Mem. Amer. Acad., N. S., vol. ii. p. 381), is called monk-fish in Maine. — *Williamson, Hist.*, vol. i. p. 157.

[1] See p. 97.

[2] "The muscle is of two sorts, — sea-muscles (in which they find pearl) and river-muscles." — *Voyages*, p. 110. See p. 37, of the present volume, for an account of "the scarlet muscle," which . . . yieldeth a perfect purple or scarlet juice; dyeing linnen so that no washing will wear it out," &c. This could scarcely have been a *Purpura* or *Buccinum*.

[3] See *Voyages*, p. 110. "The oysters be great ones," says Wood; "in form of a shoe-horn: some be a foot long. These breed on certain banks that are bare

Porpuife or *Porpifs*, *Molcbut*, *Sca Hog*, *Sus Marinus*, *Turfion*.

Prieft Fifh or *Sca Prieft*.

Prawn or *Crangone*.

Punger.

Patella.

Powt, the *Feathered Fifh*, or *Fork Fifh*.

River Powt.

Purfefifh, or *Indian Reverfus*, like an *Eel;* having a Skin on the hinder part of her Head, like a Purfe, with ftrings, which will open and fhut.

Parratfifh.

Purplefifh.

Porgee.

Remora, or *Suck Stone*, or *Stop Ship*.

Sea Raven.

[30] *Roch* or *Roach*.

Rochet or *Rouget*.

Ruff or *Pope*.

Sca Ram.

Salmon.[1]

Sailfifh.

---

every spring-tide."— *New-Eng. Prospect*, chap. ix. This was in the waters of Massachusetts Bay, where Higginson (New-Eng. Plantation, *l. c.*, p. 120) also speaks of their being found. The question whether the oyster is an indigenous inhabitant of our bay, or only an introduced stranger, is considered by Dr. Gould (Report on Invert. Animals of Mass., pp. 135, 365).

[1] One of the fishes "in greatest request" among the Indians (p. 37). Wood says it "is as good as it is in England. and in great plenty in some places."— *New-Eng. Prospect*, chap. ix.

Scallope or *Venus Cockle.*
Scate, or *Ray*, or *Griftlefifh;* of which divers kinds; as
   sharp snowted Ray, Rock Ray, &c.
Shad.[1]
Shallow.
Sharpling.
Spurling.
Sculpin.
Sheepfhead.[2]
Soles, or *Tonguefifh,* or *Sea Capon,* or *Sea Partridge.*
Seal, or *Soil,* or *Zeal.*[3]
Sea Calf, and (as fome will have it) *Molebut.*
Sheathfifh.[4]
Sea Scales.
Sturgeon; of the Roe of this Fifh they make *Caviare,* or
   Cavialtie.[5]

---

[1] "The shads be bigger than the English shads, and fatter." — *Wood, l. c.*

[2] "*Taut-auog* (sheep's-heads)." So Roger Williams's Key, *l. c.*, p. 224. It is probable, therefore, that our author had the fish that we call tautog in his mind here. What is now called sheep's-head is not known in Massachusetts Bay and northward. — *Storer, l. c.*, p. 36.

[3] See p. 34; and Wood, *l. c.*, chap. ix.

[4] See p. 96. It appears to be the mollusk, the shell of which is well known as the razor-shell (*Solen ensis*, L.). — *Gould, Report*, p. 28.

[5] See p. 32. "The sturgeons be all over the country; but the best catching of them is upon the shoals of Cape Cod and in the river of Merrimack, where much is taken, pickled, and brought to England. Some of these be 12, 14, and 18 feet long." — *Wood. New-Eng. Prospect*, chap. ix. R. Williams says that "the natives, for the goodness and greatness of it, much prize it; and will neither furnish the English with so many, nor so cheap, that any great trade is like to be made of it, until the English themselves are fit to follow the fishing." — *Key, l. c.*, p. 224. It is one of Josselyn's eight fish which are in "greatest request" with the Indians (p. 37). He calls "Pechipscut" River, in Maine, "famous for multitudes of mighty large sturgeon." — *Voyages*, p. 204.

Shark or *Bunch*, several kinds.[1]

Smelt.

Snaccot.

[31] *Shrimp.*

Spyfish.

Spitefish.

Sprat.

Spungefish.

Squill.

Squid.[2]

Sunfish.

Starfish.[3]

Swordfish.

Tench.

Thornback or *Neptunes Beard.*

Thunnie, they cut the Fifh in pieces like fhingles and powder it, and this they call *Melandria.*

Sea Toad.

Tortoife, Tortcife, Tortuga, Tortiffe, Turcle or *Turtle,* of divers kinds.[4]

Trout.[5]

---

[1] See Voyages, pp. 105–6.

[2] "This fish is much used for bait to catch a cod, hacke, polluck, and the like sea-fish." — *Voyages,* p. 107. It is still so used.

[3] Described at p. 95.

[4] See p. 34 of this, and p. 109 of the Voyages, where the author says, "Of sea-turtles, there are five sorts; of land-turtles, three sorts, — one of which is a right land-turtle, that seldom or never goes into the water; the other two being the river-turtle and the pond-turtle." — See also the author's observations on sea-turtles, at p. 39 of the Voyages.

[5] "Trouts there be good store in every brook; ordinarily two and twenty inches long. Their grease is good for the piles and clifts." — *Voyages,* p. 110..

Turbut.[1]

Sea Tun.

Sea Tree.

Uraniscopus.

Ulatife or *Sawfish*, having a Saw in his Forehead three foot long, and very sharp.

Umber.

Sea Urchin.

[32) *Sea Unicorn* or *Sea Mononeros.*

Whale, many kinds.[2]

Whiting or *Merling*, the young ones are called *Weerlings* and *Mops.*

Whore.[3]

Yardfish, Asses Prick or *Shamefish.*

The Sturgeon.

The *Sturgeon*, of whose Sounds is made Isinglafs, a kind of Glew much ufed in Phyfick: This Fifh is here in great plenty, and in fome Rivers fo numerous, that it is hazardous for Canoes and the like fmall Veffels to pafs to and again, as in *Pechipfcut* River to the Eaftward.

The Cod.

The *Cod*, which is a ftaple Commodity in the Country.

---

1 See Storer's Report. p. 146.

2 See p. 35; and Voyages, p. 104. "The natives cut them in several parcel, and give and send them far and near for an acceptable present or dish." — *R. Williams. Key, l. c.,* p. 224.

3 See Voyages. p. 110. This is the common sea-egg; *Echinus granulatus,* Say. — *Gould's Rep.,* p. 344.

To ſtop Fluxes of Blood.

In the Head of this Fiſh is found a Stone, or rather a Bone, which being pulveriz'd and drank in any convenient liquor, will ſtop Womens overflowing Courſes notably: Likewiſe,

[33] *For the Stone.*

There is a Stone found in their Bellies, in a Bladder againſt their Navel, which being pulveriz'd and drank in White-wine Poſſet or Ale, is preſent Remedy for the Stone.

To heal a green Cut.

About their Fins you may find a kind of Louſe, which healeth a green Cut in ſhort time.

To reſtore them that have melted their Greaſe.

Their Livers and Sounds eaten, is a good Medicine for to reſtore them that have melted their Greaſe.

The Dogfiſh.

The *Dogfiſh*, a ravenous Fiſh.

For the Toothach.

Upon whoſe Back grows a Thorn two or three Inches long, that helps the Toothach, ſcarifying the Gums therewith.

Their Skins are good to cover Boxes and Inſtrument Caſes.

[34] *The Stingray.*

The *Stingray*, a large Fifh, of a rough Skin, good to cover Boxes and Hafts of Knives, and Rapier fticks.

The Tortous.

The *Turtle* or *Tortous*, of which there are three kinds: 1. The land *Turtle ;* they are found in dry fandy Banks, under old Houfes, and never go into the water.

For the Ptifick, Confumption, and Morbus Gallicus.

They are good for the Ptifick and Confumptions, and fome fay the *Morbus Gallicus.*

2. The River *Turtle,* which are venomous and ftink.

3. The *Turtle* that lives in Lakes and is called in *Virginia* a *Terrapine.*

The Soile.

The *Soile* or *Sea Calf*, a Creature that brings forth her young ones upon dry land, but at other times keeps in the Sea preying upon Fifh.

[35] *For Scalds and Burns, and for the Mother.*

The Oyl of it is much ufed by the *Indians*, who eat of it with their Fifh, and anoint their limbs therewith, and their Wounds and Sores: It is very good for Scalds and Burns; and the fume of it, being caft upon Coals, will bring Women out of the Mother Fits. The Hair upon

J

the young ones is white, and as foft as filk; their Skins, with the Hair on, are good to make Gloves for the Winter.

The Sperma Ceti Whale.

* The *Sperma Ceti Whale* differeth from the *Whales* that yield us Whale-bones, for the firft hath great and long Teeth, the other is nothing but Bones with Taffels hanging from their Jaws, with which they fuck in their prey.

What Sperma Ceti is.

It is not long fince a *Sperma Ceti Whale* or two were caft upon the fhore, not far from *Boflon* in the *Maffachu-fetts Bay*, which being cut into fmall pieces and boiled in Cauldrons, yielded plenty of Oyl; the Oyl put up into Hogfheads, and ftow'd into Cellars for fome time, Candies at the [36] bottom, it may be one quarter; then the Oyl is drawn off, and the Candied Stuff put up into convenient Veffels is fold for *Sperma Ceti*, and is right *Sperma Ceti*.

For Bruifes and Aches.

The Oyl that was drawn off Candies again and again, if well ordered; and is admirable for Bruifes and Aches.

What Ambergreece is.

Now you muft underftand this *Whale* feeds upon *Ambergreece*, as is apparent, finding it in the *Whales* Maw in great quantity, but altered and excrementitious: I conceive that *Ambergreece* is no other than a kind of Mufhroom growing at the bottom of fome Seas; I was once shewed (by a Mariner) a piece of *Ambergreece* having a root to it like that of the land Mushroom, which the *Whale* breaking up, some scape his devouring Paunch, and is afterwards cast upon shore.

The Coccle.[1]

A kind of *Coccle*, of whose Shell the *Indians* make their Beads called *Wompampeag* and *Mohaicks*, the first are white, the other blew, both *Orient*, and beau[37]tified with a purple Vein. The white Beads are very good to stanch Blood.

The Scarlet Muscle.

The *Scarlet Muscle*, at *Paschatawcy* a Plantation about fifty leagues by Sea Eastward from *Boston*, in a small *Cove* called *Bakers Cove* there is found this kind of *Muscle* which hath a purple Vein, which being prickt with a Needle yieldeth a perfect purple or scarlet juice, dying Linnen so that no washing will wear it out, but keeps its lustre many years: We mark our Handkerchiefs and Shirts with it.[2]

Fish of greatest Esteem in the West Indies.

The *Indians* of *Peru* esteem of three Fishes more than any other, *viz.* the *Sea Tortcise*, the *Tubaron*, and the

---

1 See p. 24 and note.

2 Our author's account of the fishes of New England may take this of old Wood (N. E. Prospect, *l. c.*) for a tail-piece. "The chief fish for trade," says

Manate,[1] or *Sea Cow;* but in *New-England* the *Indians* have in greateſt requeſt, the *Baſs*, the *Sturgeon*, the *Salmon*, the *Lamprey*, the *Eel*, the *Froſt-fiſh*, the *Lobſter* and the *Clam*.

---

[38] Fourthly, Of Serpents, and Inſects,[2]

The Pond Frog.[3]

THe Pond *Frog*, which chirp in the Spring like *Sparows*, and croke like Toads in Autumn: Some of theſe when they ſet upon their breech are a Foot high;

---

he, "is a cod; but, for the use of the country, there is all manner of fish, as followeth : —

    "The king of waters, — the sea-shouldering Whale;
    The snuffing Grampus, with the oily seal;
    The storm-presaging Porpus, Herring-hog;
    Line-shearing Shark, the Cat-fish, and Sea-dog;
    The scale-fenced Sturgeon; wry-mouthed Hollibut;
    The flouncing Salmon, Codfish, Greedigut;
    Cole, Haddick, Hake, the Thornback, and the Scate,
    (Whose slimy outside makes him seld' in date;)
    The stately Bass, old Neptune's fleeting post,
    That tides it out and in from sea to coast;
    Consorting Herrings, and the bony Shad;
    Big-bellied Alewives; Mackrels richly clad
    With rainbow-colour, the Frost-fish and the Smelt,
    As good as ever Lady Gustus felt;
    The spotted Lamprons; Eels; the Lamperies,
    That seek fresh-water brooks with Argus-eyes:
    These watery villagers, with thousands more,
    Do pass and repass near the verdant shore."

  [1] See p. 97.

  [2] The account in the Voyages (pp. 114-23) is better; and Wood's, in New-England's Prospect, chap. xi. (to which last, Josselyn was possibly indebted), far better.

  [3] See "the generating of these creatures," in Voyages, p. 119. "Here, like-

the *Indians* will tell you, that up in the Country there are Pond *Frogs* as big as a Child of a year old.

For Burns, Scalds, and Inflammations.

They are of a gliftering brafs colour, and very fat, which is excellent for Burns and Scaldings, to take out the Fire, and heal them, leaving no Scar; and is alfo very good to take away any Inflammation.

The Rattle Snake.[1]

The *Rattle Snake*, who poyfons with a Vapour that comes thorough two crooked Fangs in their Mouth; the hollow of thefe Fangs are as black as Ink: The *Indians*, when weary with travelling, will [39] take them up with their bare hands, laying hold with one hand behind their Head, with the other taking hold of their Tail, and, with their teeth tear off the Skin of their backs, and feed upon them alive; which they fay refrefheth them.

For frozen Limbs, Aches, and Bruifes.

They have Leafs of Fat in their Bellies, which is ex-cellent to annoint frozen Limbs, and for Aches ·and

---

wise," says Wood, "be great store of frogs, which, in the spring, do chirp and whistle like a bird; and, at the latter end of summer, croak like our English frogs." — *N. Eng. Prospect, l. c.* In his Voyages, Josselyn speaks (as Wood had done) of the tree-toad, and also of another kind of toad; and of "the eft, or swift, . . . a most beautiful creature to look upon; being larger than ours, and painted with glorious colours: but I lik'd him never the better for it" (p. 119).

[1] Wood's account (New-Eng. Prospect, *l. c.*) is worth comparing with Higgin-son's (New-England's Plantation, *l. c.*) and with Josselyn's, both here and at pp.

Bruifes wondrous foveraign.   Their Hearts fwallowed
frefh, is a good Antidote againft their Venome, and their
Liver (the Gall taken out) bruifed and applied to their
Bitings is a prefent Remedy.

---

23 and 114 of the Voyages. Wood justly says of this "most poisonous and dangerous creature," that it is "nothing so bad as the report goes of him. . . . He is
naturally," he continues, "the most sleepy and unnimble creature that lives;
never offering to leap or bite any man, if he be not trodden on first: and it is
their desire, in hot weather, to lie in paths where the sun may shine on them;
where they will sleep so soundly, that I have known four men to stride over
them, and never awake her. . . . Five or six men," he adds, "have been bitten
by them; which, by using of snake-weed" (compare the preface to this, p. 119),
"were all cured; never any yet losing his life by them. Cows have been bitten;
but, being cut in divers places, and this weed thrust into their flesh, were cured.
I never heard of any beast that was yet lost by any of them, saving one mare"
(l. c.). Of other serpents, Wood mentions the black snake; and Josselyn, in his
Voyages (l. c.), speaks of "infinite numbers, of various colours;" and especially
of "one sort that exceeds all the rest; and that is the checkquered snake, having
as many colours within the checkquers shadowing one another as there are in a
rainbow." He says again, "The water-snake will be as big about the belly as the
calf of a man's leg" which is, perhaps, the water-adder. Josselyn adds, "I never
heard of any mischief that snakes did" (l. c.); and so Wood: "Neither doth any
other kind of snakes" (the rattle-snake always excepted, as no doubt dangerous
when trodden on) "molest either man or beast." There are perhaps no worse
prejudices in common life, than those which breed cruelty. In the Voyages (p.
23), our author makes mention "of a sea-serpent, or snake, that lay quoiled up
like a cable upon a rock at Cape Ann. A boat passing by with English aboard,
and two Indians, they would have shot the serpent: but the Indians disswaded
them; saying, that, if he were not kill'd outright, they would be all in danger of
their lives." This was from "some neighbouring gentlemen in our house, who
came to welcome me into the countrey;" and it seems, that, "amongst variety of
discourse, they told me also of a young lyon (not long before) killed at Piscataway by an Indian;" which, indeed, was possibly not without foundation. And
as to the serpent, compare a Report of a Committee of the Linnæan Society of
New England relative to a large marine animal, supposed to be a serpent, seen
near Cape Ann, Mass., in August, 1817 (Boston, 1817); which contains also a
full account of a smaller animal—supposed not to differ, even in species, from
the large—which was taken on the rocks of Cape Ann.—See also Storer, Report
on the Reptiles of Mass.; Supplement, p. 410.

Of Insects.[1]

A Bug.

THere is a certain kind of *Bug* like a *Beetle*, but of a glittering brafs colour, with four ftrong Tinfel Wings; their Bodies are full of Corruption or white Matter like a Maggot; being dead, and kept awhile, they will ftench odioufly; they beat the *Humming Birds* from the Flowers.

[40] *The Wafp.*

The *Wafps* in this Countrey are pied, black and white, breed in Hives made like a great Pine Apple, their entrance is at the lower end, the whole Hive is of an Afh Colour, but of what matter its made no man knows; wax it is not, neither will it melt nor fry, but will take fire fuddenly like Tinder: this they faften to a Bow, or build it round about a low Bufh, a Foot from the ground.

The flying Gloworm.

The flying *Gloworm*, flying in dark Summer Nights like fparks of Fire in great number; they are common liewife, in *Palcftina*.

---

[1] The author continues his entomological observations, in his Voyages, p. 115; and the account is fuller than Wood's; *New-England's Prospect*, chap. xi.

[41] Fifthly, Of Plants.

AND

1. *Of such Plants as are common with us in* ENGLAND.

H *Edghog-grass.*[1]
      Mattweed.[2]
Cats-tail.[3]

---

[1] Gerard by Johnson, p. 17, — *Carex flava*, L.; the first species of this genus indicated in North America, and common also to Europe. There is no doubt of the reference, taking Josselyn's name to be meant for specific, and to refer to Gerard's first figure with the same name. But it is certainly possible that our author had in view only a general reference to Gerard's fourteenth chapter, "Of Hedgehog Grasse," which brings together plants of very different genera; and, in this case, his name is of little account. Cutler (Account of Indig. Veg., *l. c.*, 1785) mentions three genera of *Cyperaceæ*, but not *Carex;* nor did he ever publish that description of our true *Gramineæ* "and other native grasses," which, he says (*l. c.*, p. 407), "may be the subject of another paper." The first edition of Bigelow's Florula Bostoniensis (1814) has seven species of *Carex*, which are increased to seventeen in the second edition (1824); the list embracing the most common and conspicuous forms. The genus has since been made an object of special study, and the number of our species, in consequence, greatly increased. A list of Carices of the neighborhood of Boston, published by the present writer in 1841 (Hovey's Mag. Hort.), gives forty-seven species; and Professor Dewey's Report on the Herbaceous Plants of Massachusetts, in 1840, reckons ninety-one species within the limits of his work.

[2] Johnson's Gerard, p. 42, — English matweed, or helme (the other species being excluded, as not English, by our author's caption); which I take to be *Calamagrostis arenaria* (L.) Roth, of Gray, Man., p. 548; called sea-matweed in England, and common to Europe and America. But if the author only intended to refer to Gerard's "Chapter 34, of Mat-weed," — which is perhaps, on the whole, unlikely, — his name is of no value.

[3] Gerard, p. 46, — *Typha latifolia*, L., — common to America and Europe.

Stichwort, commonly taken here by ignorant People for *Eyebright*; it blows in *June.*[1]

Blew Flower-de-luce; the roots are not knobby, but long and ftreight, and very white, with a multitude of ftrings.[2]

To provoke Vomit and for Bruifes.

It is excellent for to provoke Vomiting, and for Bruifes on the Feet or Face. They Flower in *June*, and grow upon dry fandy Hills as well as in low wet Grounds.

Yellow baftard Daffodill; it flowereth in *May*, the green leaves are fpotted with black fpots.[3]

Dogftones, a kind of *Satyrion*, whereof there are feveral kinds groweth in our Salt Marfhes.[4]

[42] To procure Love.

I once took notice of a wanton Womans compounding the folid Roots of this Plant with Wine, for an Amorous Cup; which wrought the defired effect.

---

[1] Gerard, p. 47, — *Stellaria graminea*, L.; for which our author mistook, as did Cutler a century after, the nearly akin *S. longifolia*, Muhl.

[2] Appears not to be meant for a specific reference to any of Gerard's species; but only an indication of the genus, with the single distinguishing character of color, which was enough to separate the New-England plants from the only British one referred by Gerard to Iris. Both of our blue-flags are peculiar to the country.

[3] Not one of Gerard's bastard daffodils, but his dog's-tooth, p. 204 (*Erythronium*, L.). Our common dog's-tooth was at first taken for a variety of the European, but is now reckoned distinct.

[4] Gerard. p. 205, — *Orchis*, L., etc. It is here clear that the name is used only in a general way. The second name (*Satyrion*), perhaps, however, makes our author's notion a little more definite, and permits us to refer the plants he had probably in view to species of *Platanthera*, Rich. (Gray, Man., p. 444), of which only one is certainly known to be common to us and Europe.

K

Watercreffes.[1]

Red Lillies grow all over the Country innumerably amongst the small Bushes, and flower in *June.*[2]

Wild Sorrel.[3]

Adders Tongue comes not up till *June*; I have found it upon dry hilly grounds, in places where the water hath stood all Winter, in *August*, and did then make Oyntment of the Herb new gathered; the fairest Leaves grow amongst short *Hawthorn* Bushes, that are plentifully growing in such hollow places.[4]

One Blade.[5]

Lilly Convallie, with the yellow Flowers grows upon rocky banks by the Sea.[6]

---

[1] Gerard, em. p. 257, — *Nasturtium officinale*, L. Reckoned also by Cutler, and indeed naturalized in some parts of the country (Gray, Man., p. 30); but our author had probably *N. palustre*, DC. (marsh-cress), if any thing of this genus, and not rather *Cardamine hirsuta*, L. (hairy lady's smock), in his mind. Both the last are common to us and Europe. — *Gray, l. c.*

[2] Gerard, p. 192. *Lilium bulbiferum* (the garden red lily) is meant; for which our author mistook our own red lily (*L. Philadelphicum*, L.).

[3] Of the two plants, — either of which may possibly have been in view of the author here, — the sorrell du bois, or white wood-sorrel of Gerard, p. 1101 (*Oxalis acetosella*, L.) which is truly common to Europe and America, and the sheep's sorrel (Gerard, p. 397, — *Rumex acetosella*, L.), which inhabits, indeed, the whole northern hemisphere, but is taken by Dr. Gray to be a naturalized weed here, I incline to think the latter less likely to have escaped Josselyn's attention than the former, and to be what he means to say appeared to him as native, in 1671. For the yellow wood-sorrel, see farther on.

[4] Gerard, em., p. 404, — *Ophioglossum vulgatum*, L.; common to us and Europe.

[5] Gerard, em., p. 409, — *Smilacina bifolia* (L.), Ker; common to us and Europe.

[6] Gerard, em., p. 410. A mistake of our author's, which can hardly be set right. The station is against the plant's having been *Smilacina trifolia* (L.), Desf. But it may be that *Clintonia borealis* (Ait.) Raf., was intended.

Water Plantane, here called *Water fuck-leaves*.[1]

For Burns and Scalds, and to draw Water out of fwell'd Legs.

It is much ufed for Burns and Scalds, and to draw water out of fwell'd Legs. *Bears* feed much upon this Plant, fo do the *Moofe Deer*.

[43] *Sea Plantane*, three kinds.[2]

Small-water Archer.[3]

Autumn Bell Flower.[4]

White Hellibore, which is the firft Plant that fprings up in this Country, and the firft that withers; it grows in deep black Mould and Wet, in fuch abundance, that you may in a fmall compafs gather whole Cart-loads of it.[5]

---

[1] *Alisma plantago*, L., common to Europe and America; "called, in New England, water suck-leaves and scurvie-leaves. You must lay them whole to the leggs to draw out water between the skin and the flesh." — *Josselyn's Voyages*, p. 80. As to its medicinal properties, see Gerard, p. 419; and Wood and Bache, Dispens., p. 1293.

[2] *Plantago maritima*, L. (Gerard, p. 423), a native of Europe and America, is our only sea-plantain. One of the others was probably *Triglochin*.

[3] *Sagittaria sagittifolia*, L. (now called arrowhead), common to Europe and America; though here passing into some varieties which are unknown in the European Floras.

[4] *Gentiana saponaria*, L., peculiar to America, but nearly akin to the European *G. pneumonanthe*, L., which our author intended. — *Johnson's Gerard*, edit. cit., p. 438.

[5] The plant is green hellebore (*Veratrum viride*, Ait.); so near, indeed, to the white hellebore (*V. album*, L.) of Europe, that it was taken for it by Michaux. In his Voyages, the author, after speaking of the use of opium by the Turks, says, "The English in New England take white hellebore, which operates as fairly with them as with the Indians," &c. (p. 60); and see p. 76, further.

Wounds and Aches Cured by the Indians. *For the Tooth-ach. For Herpes milliares.*

The *Indians* Cure their Wounds with it, annointing the Wound firſt with Raccoons greeſe, or Wild-Cats greeſe, and ſtrewing upon it the powder of the Roots; and for Aches they ſcarifie the grieved part, and annoint it with one of the foreſaid Oyls, then ſtrew upon it the powder: The powder of the Root put into a hollow Tooth, is good for the Tooth-ach: The Root ſliced thin and boyled in Vineager, is very good againſt *Herpes Milliaris.*

Arſmart, both kinds.[1]

Spurge Time, it grows upon dry ſandy Sea Banks, and is very like to *Rupter-wort*, it is full of Milk.[2]

Rupter-wort, with the white flower.[3]

---

[1] *Polygonum lapathifolium*, L. (*Hydropiper* of Gerard, p. 445), — for which, perhaps, *P. hydropiper*, L., was mistaken, — and *P. Persicaria*, L. (*Persicaria maculosa* of Gerard, *l. c.*), are what the author means; being the two sorts figured by Gerard himself. The third, added by Johnson, is unknown in this country; and the fourth belongs to a very different genus. *P. Persicaria* is marked as introduced in the late Mr. Oakes's catalogue of the plants of Vermont; and both this and *P. hydropiper* are considered to be naturalized weeds by Dr. Gray (Man., p. 373). Josselyn's testimony as to the former, as appearing to him to be native in 1671, is therefore not without interest; and possibly it is not quite worthless as to the latter.

[2] *Chamæsyce*, or spurge-time, of Gerard (*edit. cit.*, p. 504), is *Euphorbia chamæsyce*, L., a species belonging to the Eastern continent; for which Sloane (*cit. L. Sp. Pl. in loco*) appears to have mistaken our *Euphorbia maculata*, L.; while Plukenet (*Alm.* 372, *cit. L.*) recognizes the affinity of the same plants, calling the latter *Chamæsyce altera Virginiana.* Josselyn's spurge-time may be *E. maculata;* but quite possibly, taking the station which he gives into the account, *E. polygonifolia*, L.

[3] There are " several sorts of spurge," according to the Voyages (p. 78); of which this, which I cannot specifically refer, is possibly one.

Jagged *Rofe-penny-wort*.[1]

[44] *Soda bariglia*, or *maffacote*, the Afhes of *Soda*, of which they make Glaffes.

Glafs-wort, here called *Berrelia*, it grows abundantly in Salt Marfhes.[2]

St. John's-Wort.[3]

St. Peter's-Wort.[4]

---

[1] To this species of *Saxifraga*, L., unknown to our *Flora* (Gerard, p. 528), our author, with little doubt, referred the pretty *S. Virginiensis*, Michx. — See p. 58 of this, note.

[2] Gerard, em., p. 535, — *Salicornia herbacea*, L. But Linnæus referred one of Clayton's Virginia specimens (the rest he did not distinguish from *S. herbacea*) to a variety, β. *Virginica* (which he took to be also European; *Sp. Pl.*), and afterwards raised this to a species, as *S. Virginica*, *Syst. Nat.*, vol. ii. p. 52, Willd. *Sp. Pl.*, vol. i. p. 25. To this the more common glasswort of our salt marshes is to be referred; and we possess, beside, a still better representative of the European plant in *S. mucronata*, Bigel. (*Fl. Bost.*, edit. 2, p. 2), which may perhaps best be taken for a peculiar variety (*S. herbacea*, β. *mucronata*, articulorum dentibus squamisque mucronatis, *Enum. Pl. Cantab.*, Ms.; and *S. Virginica* may well be another) of a species common to us and Europe. It is certain that we have plants strictly common to American and European Floras, in which the differences referable to difference of atmospheric and other like conditions are either not apparent or of no account; and it is possible that there are yet other species, now considered peculiar to America, which only differ from older European species in those characters — whether of exuberance mostly, or also of impoverishment — in which an American variety of a plant, common to America and Europe, might beforehand be expected to differ from an European state of the same. "Linnæus ut Tournefortii errores corrigeret, varietates nimis contraxit." — *Link, Phil. Bot.*, p. 222.

[3] *Hypericum perforatum*, L. ("*Hypericum, S. John's-wort*; in shops, *Perforata*." — *Gerard, edit. cit.*, p. 539). The species is considered to have been introduced, by most American authors; and it is possible that Josselyn had *H. corymbosum*, Muhl., in his mind.

[4] *Hypericum quadrangulum*, L. (Gerard, p. 542); for which our author doubtless mistook *H. mutilum*, L. (*H. parviflorum*, Willd.), a species peculiar to America; to which Cutler's *H. quadrangulum* (Account of Indig. Veg., *l. c.*, p. 474) is probably also to be referred.

Speed-well Chick-weed.[1]
Male fluellin, or *Speed-well.*[2]
Upright Peniroyal.[3]
Wild-Mint.[4]
Cat-Mint.[5]
Egrimony.[6]
The leffer *Clot-Bur.*[7]

Water Lilly, with yellow Flowers, the *Indians* Eat the Roots, which are long a boiling, they taft like the Liver of a Sheep, the *Moofe Deer* feed much upon them, at which time the *Indians* kill them, when their heads are under water.[8]

Dragons, their leaves differ from all the kinds with us, they come up in *June.*[9]

---

[1] *Veronica arvensis,* L. (Gerard, p. 613), — a native, at present, of Europe, Asia, Northern Africa, and North America (Benth., in DC. Prodr., vol. x. p. 482); but considered to have been introduced here.

[2] *Veronica,* L. The species is perhaps *V. officinalis,* L.; which, together with *V. serpyllifolia,* L., is considered by Prof. Gray to be both indigenous and introduced here. — *Man. Bot.,* pp. 200–1.

[3] *Hedeoma pulegioides* (L.) Pers. (American pennyroyal), is doubtless meant. The specific name indicates its resemblance — in smell and taste particularly — to *Mentha pulegium,* L.; for which our author and Cutler (*l. c.,* p. 461) mistook it. But the former is peculiar to America.

[4] *Mentha aquatica,* L. *Sp. Pl.* (Gerard, p. 684); for which it is likely our author (and also Cutler, *l. c.,* p. 460) mistook *M. Canadensis,* L., Gray.

[5] *Nepeta cataria,* L. (Gerard, em., p. 682); considered by American botanists to have been introduced from Europe.

[6] *Agrimonia Eupatoria,* L. (Gerard, em., p. 712); common to America and Europe.

[7] *Xanthium strumarium,* L., Gray (Gerard, p. 809); common, as a species, to both continents; but in part, also, introduced. — *Gray, Man.,* p. 212.

[8] *Nuphar advena,* Ait., — the common American species, — is meant; and this, though resembling *N. lutea,* Sm., of Europe, is distinct from it.

[9] *Arum,* L. (Gerard, p. 381). The New-England species "differ," as our author says, "from all the kinds" in the Old World.

Violets of three kinds, the White Violet which is, fweet, but not fo ftrong as our Blew Violets; Blew Violets without fent, and a Reddifh Violet without fent; they do not blow till *June*.[1]

[45] *For ſwell'd Legs.*

Wood-bine, good for hot fwellings of the Legs, foment- ing with the decoction, and applying the *Feces* in the form of a *Cataplaſme*.[2]

Salomons-Seal, of which there is three kinds; the firſt common in *England*, the fecond, *Virginia Salomons-Seal*, and the third, differing from both, is called *Treacle Berries*, having the perfect taſt of Treacle when they are ripe; and will keep good along while; certainly a very whol- fome Berry, and medicinable.[3]

---

[1] None of the species, presumably here meant, are common to America and Europe. Our author's white violet is *Viola blanda*, Willd.

[2] All our true honeysuckles ("woodbinde, or honisuckles," — Gerard, p. 891; *Caprifolium*. Juss.) are distinct from those of Europe; but what the author meant here is uncertain.

[3] *Convallaria*, L.; *Polygonatum*, Tourn.; *Smilacina*, Desf. Many botanists have referred our smaller Solomon's seal to the nearly akin *C. multiflora* of Eu- rope; but Dr. Gray (Manual, p. 466) pronounces the former a distinct American species. The second of Josselyn's species is the "*Polygonatum Virginianum*, or Virginian's Salomon's seale" of Johnson's Gerard (p. 905), and also of Morison (Hist., *cit. L.*), and earliest described and figured by Cornuti as *P. Canadense*, &c., which is *Smilacina stellata*, (L.) Desf.; peculiar to America. The third is set down by our author, at p. 56, among the "plants proper to the country;" and Wood (New-Eng. Prospect, chap. v.) mentions it among eatable wild fruits, by the same name. It is probably *Smilacina racemosa*, (L.) Desf., — a suggestion which I owe to my friend Rev. J. L. Russell's notes upon Josselyn's plants, in Hovey's Magazine (March, April, and May, 1858); papers which were published after the manuscript of this edition had passed from the hands of the editor, — and is also confined to this continent.

* *Doves-Foot.*[1]
  Herb Robert.[1]
  Knobby Cranes Bill.[1]

For Agues.

Ravens-Claw, which flowers in *May*, and is admirable for Agues.[1]

Cinkfoil.[2]

Tormentile.[2]

Avens, with the leaf of *Mountane-Avens*, the flower and root of *Englifh Avens.*[3]

Strawberries.[4]

---

[1] *Geranium*, L. The first is *G. Carolinianum*, L., which nearly resembles Gerard's dove's-foot (p. 938); the second is *G. Robertianum*, L., common to us and Europe; and the third (Gerard, p. 940) — which cannot be *G. diffectum* — was meant, it is likely to be taken for synonymous with the fourth, or raven's-claw, — doubtless our lovely *G. maculatum*, L., which belongs to that group of species which the old botanists distinguished by the common name *Geranium batrachioides*, or crow-foot geranium, which flowers in May, and is of well-known value in medicine; and the "knobby" root, attributed to Josselyn's third kind, favors this opinion.

[2] The genus *Potentilla*, L., in general, is perhaps intended by cinque-foil; and although our author probably confounded the common and variable *Potentilla Canadensis*, L., with the nearly akin *P. reptans* and *P. verna*, L., of Europe, yet the larger part of our New-England species are, with little doubt, common to both continents. What Josselyn referred to *Tormentilla*, L., — a genus not now separated from *Potentilla*, — was probably a state of *P. Canadensis*, which resembles *P. reptans*, L., as remarked above (and was, indeed, mistaken for it by Cutler, — *l. c.*, p. 453), as this does *Tormentilla reptans*, L.

[3] *Geum strictum*, Ait., — not found in England, but European (Gray, Man., p. 116), — is indicated by the author's phrase; and see the Voyages, p. 78, for his opinion of its medicinal virtue.

[4] *Fragaria vesca*, L. (the common wood-strawberry of Europe), is native here, according to Oakes (Catal. Verm., p. 12), "especially on mountains;" and I have even gathered it, but possibly naturalized, on the woody banks of Fresh

Wild Angelica, majoris and *minoris.*[1]

Alexanders, which grow upon Rocks by the Sea fhore.[2]

[46] *Yarrow,* with the white Flower.[3]

Columbines, of a flefh colour, growing upon Rocks.[4]

Oak of Hierufalem.[5]

Pond in Cambridge. Our more common strawberry was not separated from the European by Linnæus, but is now reckoned a distinct species. "There is likewise strawberries in abundance," says Wood (New-England's Prospect, *l. c.*), — very large ones; some being two inches about. One may gather half a bushel in a forenoon." — "This berry," says Roger Williams (Key, in Hist. Coll., vol. iii. p. 221), "is the wonder of all the fruits growing naturally in those parts. It is of itself excellent; so that one of the chiefest doctors of England was wont to say, that God could have made, but God never did make, a better berry. In some parts, where the natives have planted, I have many times seen as many as would fill a good ship, within few miles' compass. The Indians bruise them in a mortar, and mix them with meal, and make strawberry-bread." Gookin also speaks of Indian-bread. — *Mass. Hist. Coll.,* vol. i. p. 150.

[1] The two plants here intended, and supposed by the author to correspond with the "wild angelica" and "great wilde angelica" of Gerard (pp. 999–1000), may perhaps be taken for the same which Cornuti (*Canad. Pl. Hist.,* pp. 196–200), thirty years before, had designated as new, — Josselyn's *Angelica sylvestris minor* being *Angelica lucida Canadensis* of Cornuti, which is *A. lucida,* L. (and probably, as the French botanist describes the fruit as "minus foliacea vulgaribus," also *Archangelica peregrina,* Nutt.); and his *Angelica sylvestris major* being *A. atropurpurea Canadensis* of Cornuti, or *A. atropurpurea,* L.

[2] *Smyrnium aureum,* L. (golden Alexanders), now separated from that genus, was mistaken, it is quite likely, for *S. olusatrum,* L. (true Alexanders), to which it bears a considerable resemblance. — *Gerard,* p. 1019.

[3] *Achillea millefolium,* L. Oakes has marked this as introduced (Catal. Vermont, p. 17): but it appeared to our author, in 1672, to be indigenous; and Dr. Gray reckons it among plants common to both hemispheres. — *Statistics of Amer. Flora,* in Am. Jour. Sci., vol. xxiii. p. 70. The author's reference is to common yarrow. — *Gerard,* p. 1072.

[4] *Aquilegia Canadensis,* L. As elsewhere, the author probably means here only that the genus is common to both continents.

[5] At p. 56, both of these are set down among the "plants proper to the country." The first, to follow Gerard (p. 1108), is *Chenopodium botrys,* L., — a native of the south of Europe, and considered as an introduced species here. It has reputation in diseases of the chest. — Wood & Bache, Dispens., p. 213. Josselyn's

L

Acharifton is an excellent Medicine for ftopping of the Lungs upon Cold, Ptifick, &c.

Oak of *Cappadocia,* both much of a nature, but Oak of *Hierufalem* is ftronger in operation; excellent for ftuffing of the Lungs upon Colds, fhortnefs of Wind, and the Ptifick; maladies that the Natives are often troubled with: I helped feveral of the *Indians* with a Drink made of two Gallons of *Moloffes wort,* (for in that part of the Country where I abode, we made our Beer of Moloffes, Water, Bran, chips of *Saffafras* Root, and a little Wormwood, well boiled,) into which I put of Oak of *Hierufalem,* Catmint, Sowthiftle, of each one handful, of *Enula Campana* Root one Ounce, Liquorice ferap'd brufed and cut in pieces, one Ounce, Saffafras Root cut into thin chips, one Ounce, Anny-feed and fweet Fennel-feed, of each one Spoonful bruifed; boil thefe in a clofe Pot, upon a foft Fire to the confumption of one Gallon, then take it off, and ftrein it gently; you may if you will [47] boil the ftreined liquor with Sugar to a Syrup, then when it is Cold, put it up into Glafs Bottles, and take thereof three or four fpoonfuls at a time, letting it run down your throat as leafurely as poffibly you can; do thus in the morning, in the Afternoon, and at Night going to Bed.

Goofe-Grafs, or *Clivers.*[1]

---

oak of Cappadocia (Gerard, p. 1108) is an American species, — *Ambrosia elatior,* L. Cutler says of it (*l. c.,* p. 489), "It has somewhat the smell of camphire. It is used in antiseptick fomentations."

[1] *Galium aparine,* L. (Gerard, *edit. cit.,* p. 1122), common to America and Europe. — Compare Gray, Man., p. 170.

Fearn.[1]

Brakes.[1]

Wood forrel, with the yellow flower.[2]

Elm.[3]

Line Tree, both kinds.[4]

A way to draw out Oyl of Akrons, or the like, &c.
Maple; of the Afhes of this Tree the *Indians* make a lye, with which they force out Oyl from Oak Akorns that is highly efteemed by the *Indians.*[5]

Dew-Grafs.[6]

Earth-Nut, which are of divers kinds, one bearing very beautiful Flowers.[7]

---

[1] The "Filix mas, or male ferne," of Gerard, *edit. cit.*, p. 1128 (for, says he, of the "divers sorts of ferne . . . there be two sorts, according to the old writers, — the male and the female; and these be properly called ferne: the others have their proper names"), is the collective designation of four species of *Afpidium*; of which all, according to Pursh, and certainly three, are natives of both continents, — *AA. cristatum, Filix mas, Filix fœmina,* and *aculeatum,* Willd. "*Filix fœmina* (female ferne, or brakes," of Gerard, *l. c.*) is *Pteris aquilina,* L.; also common to us and Europe. The other *Filices* mentioned by our author are *Ophioglossum vulgatum,* L. (p. 42); and *Adiantum pedatum,* L. (p. 55).

[2] *Oxalis corniculata,* L. (Gerard, em., p. 1202), common to Europe and America.

[3] *Ulmus,* L. There are no species common to America and Europe.

[4] See the Voyages, p. 69, where the author has it "the line-tree, with long nuts: the other kind I could never find." The former was *Tilia Americana,* L., — a species peculiar to America.

[5] See p. 48; and Voyages, p. 69. None of our species are found in Europe.

[6] The plant intended is doubtless the same with that spoken of in the Voyages, p. 80. — "*Rosa solis,* sundew, moor-grass. This plant I have seen more of than ever I saw in my whole life before in England," &c. Both our common New-England species of *Drosera* are also natives of Europe.

[7] "Differing much from those in England. One sort of them bears a most beautiful flower" (p. 56, where it is rightly placed among plants "proper to the

Fufs-Balls, very large.[1]

Mufhrooms, fome long and no bigger than ones finger, others jagged flat, round, none like our great Mufhrooms in *England,* of thefe fome are of a Scarlet colour, others a deep Yellow, *&c.*[1]

[48] Blew flowered *Pimpernel.*[2]

Noble *Liver-wort,* one fort with white flowers, the other with blew.[3]

Black-Berry.[4]

---

country "). The author refers here, doubtless, to *Apios tuberosa,* Moench. (ground-nut of New England), which was raised at Paris, from American seeds, by Vespasian Robin, and figured from his specimens by Cornuti (Canad., p. 200) in 1635; but it was celebrated, ten years earlier, in "Nova Anglia," — a curious poem by the Rev. William Morrell, who came over with Capt. Robert Gorges in 1623, and spent about a year at Weymouth and Plymouth, publishing his book in 1625 (repr. Hist. Coll., vol. i. p. 125, &c.), — as follows: —

> "Vimine gramineo nux subterranea suavis
> Serpit humi, tenui flavo sub cortice, pingui
> Et placido nucleo nivei candoris ab intra,
> Melliflua parcos hilarans dulcedine gustus,
> Donec in æstivum Phœbus conscenderit axem.
> His nucleis laute versutus vescitur Indus:
> His exempta fames segnis nostratibus omnis
> Dulcibus his vires revocantur victibus almæ."

[1] See p. 52 and Voyages (pp. 70, 81) for other notices of *Fungi;* and Voyages, p. 81, for the only mention of *Algæ.*

[2] Female pimpernell (Gerard, em., p. 617), — *Anagallis arvensis,* γ, Sm.; *A. cærulea,* Schreb., — but scarcely differing, except in color, from the scarlet pimpernel, which has long ("in clayey ground," — *Cutler, l. c.,* 1785) been an inhabitant of the coasts of Massachusetts Bay, though doubtless introduced.

[3] *Hepatica triloba,* Chaix. (*Anemone hepatica,* L.), common to Europe and America; occurring occasionally with white flowers. — *Gerard,* em., p. 1203.

[4] *Rubus,* L. The red raspberry of this country is hardly other than an American variety of the European (*R. Idæus,* var. strigosus, caule petiolis pedunculis

Dew-Berry.

Rafp-Berry, here called *Mul-berry.*

Goofe-Berries, of a deep red Colour.[1]

Haw-thorn, the Haws being as big as Services, and very good to eat, and not fo aftringent as the Haws in *England.*[2]

Toad flax.[3]

---

calyceque aculeato-hispidissimis, Enum. Pl. Agri Cantab, 1843, Ms.); upon which see Gray (Man., p. 121; and Statistics, &c., *l. c.,* p. 81). *R. triflorus,* Richards., is also very near to, and was once considered the same as, the European *R. saxatilis,* L. The rest of our New-England raspberries and blackberries appear to be specifically distinct from those of Europe. The cloud-berry, mentioned at p. 60, is there set down among plants proper to the country; and may therefore not be the true cloud-berry (Gerard, p. 1273), or *Rubus chamæmorus,* L., which is common to both continents.

[1] The New-England gooseberries are peculiar to this country. The author no doubt intends *Ribes hirtellum,* Michx. (Gray, Man., p. 137); as see further his Voyages, p. 72.

[2] *Cratægus,* L. But the species are peculiar to this country, as Josselyn implies with respect to the haws which he notices. These, no doubt, included *C. tomentosa,* L., Gray; and perhaps, also, *C. coccinea,* L. Wood says, "The white thorn affords hawes as big as an English cherry; which is esteemed above a cherry for his goodness and pleasantness to the taste."—*New-England's Prospect,* chap. v. At page 72 of his Voyages, the author mentions "a small shrub, which is very common; growing sometimes to the height of elder; bearing a berry like in shape to the fruit of the white thorn; of a pale, yellow colour at first, then red (when it is ripe, of a deep purple); of a delicate, aromatical tast, but somewhat stiptick,—which may be *Pyrus arbutifolia,* L. Higginson (New-England's Plantation, *l. c.,* p. 119) speaks of our haws almost as highly as Wood.

[3] Great toad-flax (Gerard, em., p. 550); *Linaria vulgaris,* Moench. Compare De Candolle (Geog. Bot., vol. ii. p. 716) for a sketch of the American history of this now familiar plant, which the learned author cannot trace before Bigelow's date (Fl. Bost., edit. 1) of 1814. But it is certainly Cutler's "snapdragon; . . . blossoms yellow, with a mixture of scarlet; common by roadsides in Lynn and Cambridge" (*l. c.,* 1785): though he strangely prefixes the Linnæan phrase for *Antirrhinum Canadense,* L.; and there seems no reason to doubt that Josselyn may very well have seen it in 1671.

Pellamount, or Mountain time.[1]
Moufe-car Minor.[2]

The making of Oyl of Akrons.   To ſtrengthen weak Members.   For Scall'd-heads.

There is *Oak* of three kinds, white, red and black, the white is excellent to make Canoes of, Shallopes, Ships, and other Veſſels for the Sea, and for Claw-board, and Pipe-ſtaves, the black is good to make Waynſcot of; and out of the white Oak Acorns, (which is the Acorn Bears delight to feed upon): The Natives draw an Oyl, taking the rotteneſt Maple Wood, which being burnt to aſhes, they make a ſtrong Lye therewith, wherein they boyl their white Oak-Acorns until the Oyl ſwim on the top in great quantity; this [49] they fleet off, and put into bladders to annoint their naked Limbs, which corroborates them exceedingly; they eat it likewiſe with their Meat, it is an excellent clear and ſweet Oyl: Of the Mofs that grows at the roots of the white Oak the *Indeſſes* make a ſtrong decoction, with which they help their *Papouſes* or young Childrens ſcall'd Heads.[3]

---

[1] Gerard, p. 653 (*Teucrium*, L.). The author may have intended to reckon the genus only. Our species is peculiar to this continent.

[2] The designation is uncertain. The old botanists gave the name *Auricula muris*, or mouse-ear, to species of *Myosotis*, *Draba*, *Hieracium*, and *Gnaphalium*. Josselyn's plant may most probably be *Antennaria plantaginifolia*, Hook. (mouse-ear of New England), which is very near to *A. dioica* of Europe. — *Gray, Statistics, &c., l. c.*, p. 81.

[3] *Quercus alba*, L.; *Q. rubra*, L.; and *Q. tinctoria*, Bartr. Wood's account of the oaks (New-England's Prospect, chap. v.) is similar. In his Voyages, p. 61, Josselyn gives us "the ordering of red oake for wainscot. When they have cut it

Juniper, which *Cardanus* faith is Cedar in hot Countries, and Juniper in cold Countries; it is hear very
dwarfiſh and ſhrubby, growing for the moſt part by the
Sea ſide.[1]

Willow.[2]

Spurge Lawrel, called here *Poyſon berry*, it kills the
Engliſh Cattle if they chance to feed upon it, eſpecially
Calves.[3]

Gaul, or noble Mirtle.[4]

Elder.[5]

Dwarf Elder.[6]

down and clear'd it from the branches, they pitch the body of the tree in a muddy
place in a river, with the head downward, for some time. Afterwards they draw
it out; and, when it is seasoned sufficiently, they saw it into boards for wainscot;
and it will branch out into curious works."

[1] *Juniperus communis*, L.; common to both continents. But the author did
not probably distinguish from it *J. Virginiana*, L.; which is frequent, and often
dwarfish, near the sea.

[2] *Salix*, L.; the genus only meant here, it is likely.

[3] *Daphne Laureola*, L. (Gerard, p. 1404), with which Josselyn may have
considered *Kalmia angustifolia*, L., in some sort allied. The latter has long
been known in New England as dwarf or low laurel.

[4] *Myrica Gale*, L. (Gerard, p 1414); common to Europe and America.

[5] *Sambucus*, L. Our *S. Canadensis*, L. differs very little from the common
elder of Europe, except, as our author in his Voyages says (p. 71), in being
" shrubbie," and in not having " a smell so strong." — *Cf.* DC. *Prodr.*, vol. ii. p.
322; *Gerard*, p. 1421. The other North-American elder (*S. pubens*, Michx.) is
at least equally near to the European *S. racemosa*, L., according to Prof. Gray.

[6] "There is a sort of dwarf-elder, that grows by the sea-side, that hath a red
pith. The berries of both " — that is, of this and of the true elder mentioned
above — " are smaller than English elder; not round, but corner'd." — *Voyages*,
p. 71. Gerard's dwarf-elder (p. 1425) is *Sambucus ebulus*, L. Josselyn's may
have been a *Viburnum*; for this genus was confused with *Sambucus* by the elder
botanists. Wood (New-England Prospect, chap. v.) speaks of —

" Small eldern, by the Indian fletchers sought ; " —

which was perhaps arrow-wood, or *Viburnum dentatum*, L. .

For a Cut with a Bruſe.

Alder; An *Indian* Bruiſing and Cutting of his Knee with a fall, uſed no other remedy, than Alder Bark, chewed faſting, and laid to it, which did foon heal it.[1]

To take Fire out of a Burn.

The decoction is alſo excellent to take [50] the Fire out of a Burn or Scalld.

For Wounds and Cuts.

For Wounds and Cuts make a ſtrong decoction of Bark of Alder, pour of it into the Wound, and drink thereof. *Haſel.*[2]

For ſore Mouths, falling of the Pallat.

Filberd, both with hairy husks upon the Nuts, and ſetting hollow from the Nut, and fill'd with a kind of water of an aſtringent taſte; it is very good for ſore Mouths, and falling of the Pallat, as is the whole green Nut before it comes to Kernel, burnt and pulverized. The Kernels are ſeldom without maggots in them.[2]

---

[1] *Alnus*, Tourn. One of the three New-England species (*A. incana*, Willd.) is common to Europe and America. Another (*A. serrulata*, Willd.) "bears so great a resemblance," says F. A. Michaux, to the common European alder (*A. glutinosa*, Willd.) "in its flowers, its seeds, its leaves, its wood, and its bark, as to render a separate figure unnecessary; the only difference observable between them" being "that the European species is larger, and has smaller leaves." — *Sylva*, vol. ii. p. 114. Compare Gray, Statistics, &c., *l. c.*, p. 83. *A. viridis*, our third species, is common to Europe and this country.

[2] *Corylus*, L. Our species, which are peculiar to America, are both indicated : the "filberd. . . . with hairy husks upon the nuts," being *C. rostrata*, Ait. (beaked hazel); and that "setting hollow from the nut," — that is, larger than the nut, — *C. Americana*, Wangenh. (common hazel).

The Figure of the Walnut.

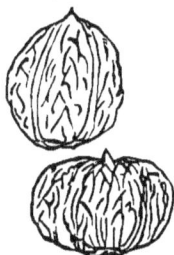

Walnut; the Nuts differ much from ours in *Europe*, they being fmooth, much like a Nutmeg in fhape, and not much bigger; fome three cornered, all of them but thinly replenifhed with Kernels.[1]

[51] *Chcfnuts*; very fweet in tafte, and may be (as

---

[1] *Carya*, Nutt. In the Voyages, p. 69, the author fpeaks of the "walnut, which is divers : some bearing square nuts; others like ours, but smaller. There is likewise black walnut, of precious use for tables, cabinets, and the like " (*Juglans nigra*, L.). " The walnut-tree," continues Josselyn, " is the toughest wood in the countrie, and therefore made use of for hoops and bowes; there being no yews there growing. In England, they made their bowes usually of witch-hasel " (that is, witch-elm, — *Ulmus montana*, Bauh., Lindl.; as see Gerard, p. 1481 : but *Carpinus*, " in Essex, is called witch-hasell," — *ib.*), ash, yew, the best of outlandish elm; but the Indians make theirs of walnut." This was hickory, and what Wood says belongs doubtless to the same. He calls it " something different from the English walnut; being a great deal more tough and more serviceable. and altogether heavy. And whereas our guns, that are stocked with English walnut, are soon broken and cracked in frost, — being a brittle wood, — we are driven to stock them new with the country walnut, which will endure all blows and weather; lasting time out of mind." After speaking favorably of the fruit, he adds (New-Eng. Profpect, chap. vi.), " There is likewise a tree, in some parts of the country, that bears a nut as big as a pear," — the butternut, doubtless (*Juglans cinerea*, L.). Josselyn has told us (p. 48) of the oil which the Indians managed to get from the acorns of the white oak. Roger Williams (Key, *l. c.*, p. 220) says our native Americans made " of these walnuts . . . an excellent oil, good for many uses. but especially for the anointing of their heads." Michaux (*Sylva*, vol. i. p. 163) says the Indians used the oil of the butternut, and also (p. 185) of the shag-bark, " to season their aliments." Williams adds (*l. c.*), " Of the chips of the walnut-tree — the bark taken off — some English in the country make excellent beer, both for taste, strength, colour, and inoffensive opening operation."

M

they ufually are) eaten raw; the *Indians* fell them to the *Englifh* for twelve pence the bufhel.[1]
Beech.[2]
Afh.[3]
Quick-beam, or *Wild-Afh.*[4]

Coals of Birch pulverized and wrought with the white of an Egg to a Salve, is a gallant Remedy for dry fcurfy Sores upon the Shins; and for Bruifed Wounds and Cuts.

Birch, white and black; the bark of Birch is ufed by the *Indians* for bruifed Wounds and Cuts, boyled very tender, and ftampt betwixt two ftones to a Plaifter, and the decoction thereof poured into the Wound; And alfo to fetch the Fire out of Burns and Scalds.[5]

---

[1] *Castanea vesca*, Gaertn.; common to Europe and America. Our chestnut is considered to differ from the European only as an American variety of a species common to both continents might be expected to. "The Indians have an art of drying their chestnuts, and so to preserve them in their barns for a dainty all the year." — *R. Williams, l. c.*

[2] Neither Wood nor R. Williams makes mention of it. The younger Michaux considered our beech distinct from the European; but Mr. Nuttall makes it only a variety of it; while Prof. Gray puts both trees in his list of "very close representative species." — *Statistics, &c., l. c.*, p. 81.

[3] *Fraxinus*, L. Our species are peculiar to this continent. I cannot account for Wood's saying, "It is different from the ash of England; being brittle and good for little, unless that walnut is used for it." — *New-Eng. Prospect*, chap. vi.

[4] *Sorbus*, L. (Gerard, p. 1473). Our mountain-ash (*S. Americana*, Willd.) is quite near to the quicken, or mountain-ash of the north of Europe.(*S. aucuparia*, L.); but hardly, perhaps, to be reduced to an American variety of it, as the elder Michaux (*Fl. Amer.*, vol. i. p. 290) proposed. Compare Gray, Statistics, &c., *l. c.*, p. 82.

[5] Except the small white birch (*B. populifolia*, Ait.), which Mr. Spach reduces to a variety of the European *B. alba*, L.. — in which he is sustained by Prof. Gray (*Man.*, p. 411), — and the dwarf-birch (*B. nana*, L.) of our alpine regions, all our

Poplar, but differing in leaf.[1]

Plumb Tree, feveral kinds, bearing fome long, round, white, yellow, red, and black Plums; all differing in their Fruit from thofe in *England*.[2]

Wild Purcelane.[3]

Wood-wax, wherewith they dye many pretty Colours.[4]

---

species are peculiar to this continent. — See the author's Voyages, p. 69, for another mention of the birches.

[1] *Populus*, L. Our species are peculiar to the country, as the author's remark suggests. Wood (*l. c.*) notices "the ever-trembling asps."

[2] "The plumbs of the country be better for plumbs than the cherries be for cherries. They be black and yellow; about the bigness of damsons; of a reasonable good taste." — *New-Eng. Prospect*, chap. v. *Prunus maritima*, Wangenh. (beech-plum), and *P. Americana*, Marsh. (wild yellow plum), are no doubt here intended; as also, it is likely, by Josselyn, who, it is evident, in this place had only the genus in mind as "common with us in England." — See p. 61 for the author's mention of the "wild cherry."

[3] *Portulaca oleracea*, L. (Gerard, p. 521). "In cornfields. It is eaten as a pot-herb, and esteemed by some as little inferior to asparagus." — *Cutler; Account of Indigenous Vegetables* (1785), *l. c.*, p. 447. Considered to have been introduced here; but our author enables us to carry back the date of its introduction, without reasonable doubt, to the first settlement of the country. "Purslain, Mr. Glover says, is also very common in Virginia, and troublesome too, to the tobacco-planters." Sir Philip Skippon to Ray, Feb. 11, 1675–6, in Ray Society's Corresp. of John Ray, p. 121. Mr. Nuttall regarded the species as indigenous on the plains of the Missouri; but this plant, "too closely resembling the common purslane," according to Prof. Gray (Man., p. 64), has been separated as specifically distinct by Dr. Engelmann.

[4] *Genista tinctoria*, L. (*Genistella tinctoria*, — greenweed, or dyers' weed; Gerard, p. 1316). "We shall not need to speake of the use that diers make thereof," says the latter. Our author could hardly have been mistaken about so well-known a plant as this; which he probably met with in one of his visits to the neighborhood of Boston, — long the only American station for it. There is a tradition that it was introduced here by Gov. Endicott; which may have been some forty years before Josselyn finished his herborizing, — enough to account for its naturalization then. It was long confined to Salem ("pastures between New Mills and Salem." — *Cutler, l. c.*, 1785); but occurred to me sparingly, in 1841, on the shores of Cambridge Bay, and also on roadsides in Old Cambridge. "Woad-seed" is set down, in a memorandum of the Governor and Company of

Red and black *Currans*.[1]

[52] *For the Gout, or any Ach.*

Spunck, an excrefcence growing out of black Birch, the *Indians* ufe it for Touchwood; and therewith they help the *Sciatica*, or Gout of the Hip, or any great Ach, burning the Patient with it in two or three places upon the Thigh, and upon certain Veins.[2]

Massachusetts Bay, before February, 1628, to be sent to New England (Mass. Col. Rec., vol. i. p. 24); and though *Isatis tinctoria*, L., is true woad, *Reseda luteola*, L. (wold, or weld), and our *Genista* (woadwaxen), have, it is said (Rees's Cycl., *in loco*), been known "in English herbals under that name."

[1] "Current-bushes are of two kinds, — red and black. The black currents, which are larger than the red, . . . are reasonable pleasant in eating." — *Voyages*, p. 72. Our black currant is *Ribes floridum*, Herit., — considered by Linnæus (Sp. Pl., p. 291) only a variety of *R. nigrum*, L., the true black currant of the gardens; and our red currant, which I have gathered in the White Mountains, — far below the region of *R. rigens*, Michx., the more common red currant there, — appears to be undistinguishable from *R. rubrum*, L. (the red currant of gardens); unless, possibly, as an American variety of it. This is probably *R. albinervium*, Michx. (Fl., vol. i. p. 110; Pursh, Fl., vol. i. p. 163).

[2] *Polyporus*, Mich., sp. — In his Voyages, p. 70, the author speaks of "a stately tree growing here and there in valleys, not like to any trees in Europe; having a smooth bark, of a dark-brown colour, the leaves like great maple in England called sycamor; but larger," — which may be *Platanus occidentalis*, L. (button-wood). And Wood enables us to add one more to this early account of the genera of plants, which we possess, common to the Old World. He tells us (New-England's Prospect, chap. v.) "the hornbound tree is a tough kind of wood, that requires so much pains in riving as is almost incredible; being the best to make bowls and dishes, not being subject to crack or leak. This tree growing with broad-spread arms, the vines twist their curling branches about them; which vines afford great store of grapes," &c. This was our American hornbeam (*Carpinus Americana*, L.). And the same author again alludes to it, in verse, as —

"The horn-bound tree, that to be cloven scorns;
Which from the tender vine oft takes his spouse,
Who twines embracing arms about his boughs."

2. *Of fuch Plants as are proper to the Country.*

To ripen any Impoftume or Swelling. For fore Mouths.
The New-Englands ftanding Difh. ✳

INdian Wheat, of which there is three forts, yellow, red, and blew; the blew is commonly Ripe before the other a Month: Five or Six Grains of *Indian* Wheat hath produced in one year 600. It is hotter than our Wheat and clammy; excellent in *Cataplafms* to ripen any Swelling or impoftume. The decoction of the blew Corn, is good to wafh fore Mouths with: It is light of digeftion, and the *Englifh* make a kind of Loblolly of it [53] to eat with Milk, which they call *Sampe*; they beat it in a Morter, and fift the flower out of it: the remainder they call *Hommincy*, which they put into a Pot of two or three Gallons, with Water, and boyl it upon a gentle Fire till it be like a Hafty Pudden; they put of this into Milk, and fo eat it. Their Bread alfo they make of the *Hommincy* fo boiled, and mix their Flower with it, caft it into a deep Bafon in which they form the Loaf, and then turn it out upon the Peel, and prefently put it into the Oven before it fpreads abroad; the Flower makes excellent Puddens.[1]

A pleasant enough illustration of what taught classical husbandry, — "*ulmis adjungere vites.*"— *Georg.*, i. 2.

[1] See also the Voyages, p. 73. "It is almost incredible," says Higginson (New-England's Plantation, *l. c.*, p. 118), "what great gaine some of our English planters have had by our Indian corne. Credible persons have assured me, — and the partie himselfe avouched the truth of it to me, — that, of the setting of

Baftard Calamus Aromaticus, agrees with the defcription, but is not barren; they flower in *July*, and grow in
wet places, as about the brinks of Ponds.[1]

To keep the Feet warm.

The *English* make ufe of the Leaves to keep their Feet
warm. There is a little Beaft called a *Mufkquafh*, that
liveth in fmall Houfes in the Ponds, like Mole Hills, that
feed upon thefe Plants. Their Cods fent as fweet and as
ftrong as Musk, and will laft along time handfomly
wrap'd up in Cotton wool; they are very good to lay
amongft Cloaths. *May* is the beft [54] time to kill them,
for then their Cods fent ftrongeft.

---

thirteen gallons of corne, hee hath had encrease of it 52 hogsheads; every hogs-
head holding seven bushels, of London measure: and every bushell was by him
sold and trusted to the Indians for so much beaver as was worth 18 shillings.
And so, of this 13 gallons of corne, which was worth 6 shillings 8 pence, he made
about 327 pounds of it the yeere following. as by reckoning will appeare; where
you may see how God blessed husbandry in this land. There is not such greate
and plentifull eares of corne, I suppose, any where else to bee found but in this
countrey; because, also of varietie of colours, — as red, blew, and yellow, &c.;
and of one corne there springeth four or five hundred." Roger Williams (Key,
l. c., pp. 208, 221) has some interesting particulars of the Indian use of their corn.
According to him, the Indian *msickquatash* (that is succotash, as we call it now)
was "boiled corn whole," and "*nawsaump*, a kind of meal pottage unparched.
From this the English call their samp; which is the Indian corn beaten and
boiled, and eaten, hot or cold; with milk or butter, — which are mercies beyond
the natives' plain water, and which is a dish exceeding wholesome for the English bodies.

[1] *Acorus Calamus*, L.; common to Europe and America. In his Voyages, p.
77, the author drops properly, in mentioning this, the injurious prefix. It seems
that our New-England forefathers used the leaves to cover their cold floors, as
they had used rushes at home; and. according to Sir W. J. Hooker (Br. Fl., vol.
i. p. 159), the pleasant smell of the plant has recommended it, in like manner,
"for strewing on the floor of the cathedral at Norwich, on festival days."

Wild-Leekes, which the *Indians* ufe much to eat with their fifh.[1]

A Plant like *Knavers-Muftard*, called *New-England* Muftard.[2]

Mountain-Lillies, bearing many yellow Flowers, turning up their Leaves like the *Martigon*, or *Turks* Cap, fpotted with fmall fpots as deep as Safforn, they Flower in *July*.[3]

One Berry, or Herb *True Love*. See the Figure.[4]

Tobacco, there is not much of it Planted in *New-England*. The *Indians* make ufe of a fmall kind with fhort round leaves called *Pooke*.[5]

---

[1] *Allium Canadense*, L., probably. — See also p. 55, note 4.

[2] "Knaves'-mustard (for that it is too bad for honest men)." — *Gerard*, p. 262. The "New-England mustard," which was like it, may be *Lepidium Virginicum*, L.; which. having "a taste like common garden-cress, or peppergrass" (Bigel., Fl. Bost., *in loco*), perhaps attracted the first settlers.

[3] The "many flowers," with reflexed sepals, perhaps refer this to our noble American Turk's-cap (*Lilium superbum*, L.), rather than to the yellow lily (*L. Canadense*, L.).

[4] See p. 81.

[5] "They take their *wuttammauog*. — that is, a weak tobacco, — which the men plant themselves, very frequently. Yet I never see any take so excessively as I have seen men in Europe; and yet excess were more tolerable in them, because they want the refreshing of beer and wine, which God had vouchsafed Europe." — *R. Williams, Key, l. c.*, p. 213. And, in another place, the same writer says that tobacco is "commonly the only plant which men labour in" (he is speaking of the Indians); "the women managing all the rest" (p. 208). Wood, in his list of Indian words (New-Eng. Prospect, *ad ult.*), spells the Indian word, above given. *ottommaocke*, — (perhaps both are comparable with "*wuttahimneash*, strawberries" (Williams, *l. c.*, p. 220), and "*weetimoquat*, it smells sweet" (Vocab. of Narraganset Lang., in Hist. Coll., vol. v. p. 82); *og, ock*, and *ash*, being all plural terminations; between which and "the noun in the singular one or more consonants or vowels are frequently interspersed" (*ibid.*, vol. iii. p. 222, note); and *oquat*, from the context, the verbal; and the root appearing possibly the same). — and also defines it as tobacco. There is much other testimony that the New-England savages were found using "tobacco" (as Mourt's Relation, *l. c.*,

For Burns and Scalds.

With a ftrong deco&tion of Tobacco they Cure Burns
and Scalds, boiling it in Water from a Quart to a Pint,
then wafh the Sore therewith, and ftrew on the powder of
dryed Tobacco.

Hollow Leaved Lavender, is a Plant that grows in falt
Marfhes overgrown with Mofs, with one ftraight ftalk
about the bignefs of an Oat ftraw, better than a Cubit
high; upon the top ftandeth one [55] fantaftical Flower,
the Leaves grow clofe from the root, in fhape like a Tankard, hollow, tough, and alwayes full of Water, the

---

p. 230; and Winslow's Relation, *l. c.*, p. 253) ; but our author's text, above, ap-
pears· to distinguish the true herb, "not much planted," from "a small kind
called *pooke*," which "the Indians make use of." And again, more clearly, in
his Voyages. we have to the same effect: "the Indians in New England use a
small, round-leafed tobacco, called by them or the fishermen *poke*. It is odious
to the English. . . . Of marchantable . . . tobacco, . . . there is little of it
planted in New England; neither have they" (both clauses appear to refer to the
English) "learned the right way of curing of it." This "marchantable tobacco"
was no doubt mainly *Nicotiana tabacum*, L.; but the other kind, the weak tobacco,"—cultivated, as Williams tells us, by the Indians, and recognized as
tobacco by the English,—was not, as Wood says (N. E. Prospe&, *l. c.*), colt's-
foot, but *Nicotiana rustica*, L. (the yellow henbane of Gerard's Herbal, p. 356),
well known to have been long in cultivation among the American savages, and
now a naturalized relic of that cultivation in various parts of the United States.
The name, *poke*, or *pooke*,—if it be, as is supposable, the same with "*puck*,
smoke," of the Narraganset vocabulary of R. Williams (Hist. Coll., vol. v. p. 84),
—was perhaps always indefinite, and, since Cutler's day, has been applied in
New England to the green hellebore (*Veratrum viride*, Ait.); but this was not, it
is evident, the poke of the first settlers. The name is also given to *Phytolacca
decandra*, L. (the *skoke* of Cutler), and the hellebore apparently distinguished
from this as Indian poke; but the application of the name to the former, at least,
probably had its origin among the whites.

Root is made up of many fmall ftrings, growing only in the Mofs, and not in the Earth, the whole Plant comes to its perfection in *Auguft*, and then it has Leaves, Stalks,

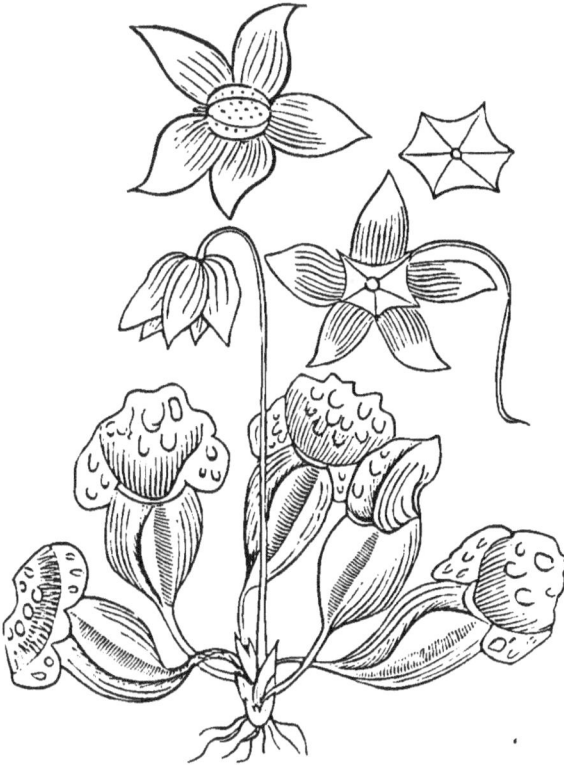

Hollow Leaved Lavender.

and Flowers as red as blood, excepting the Flower which hath fome yellow admixt.　I wonder where the

N

knowledge of this Plant hath flept all this while, *i. e.* above Forty Years.[1]

For all manner of Fluxes.

It is excellent for all manner of Fluxes.
Live for ever, a kind of *Cud-weed*.[2]
Tree Primerofe, taken by the Ignorant for *Scabious*.[3]
A Solar Plant, as fome will have it.

---

[1] The figure sufficiently exhibits *Sarracenia purpurea*, L.

[2] "Live-for-ever. It is a kind of cud-weed. . . . It growes now plentifully in our English gardens. . . . The fishermen, when they want" (that is, lack) " tobacco, take this herb; being cut and dryed."— *Voyages*, p. 78; where the author adds the peculiar medicinal virtues of the plant, which are the same as those assigned by Gerard (p. 644) to the genus. Compare, as to this, Wood and Bache, Dispens., p. 1334. The species intended by Josselyn is our everlasting (*Antennaria margaritacea* (L.) Br.), described by Gerard, and figured by Johnson in his edition of the former (p. 641), and first published by Clusius (*Gnaphalium Americanum*, Rar. Pl. Hist., vol. i. p. 327) in 1601. Clusius had it from England, says Johnson. The dried herb, used by the fishermen instead of tobacco, and no doubt called by them *poke*, may have been mistaken by Wood for colt's-foot, the leaves of which were " smoked by the ancients in pulmonary complaints; . . . and, in some parts of Germany, are at the present time said to be substituted for tobacco."— *Wood and Bache, Dispens.*, p. 1401. *Cornus sericea*, L.,— "called by the natives squaw-bush" (Williamson's Hist. Maine, vol. i. p. 125), and by the western Indians *kinnikinnik* (Gray, Man., p. 161); furnished, in its inner bark (the medicinal properties of which, see especially Rees's Cycl., Amer. ed., *in loco*), a substitute for *Nicotiana*, — very widely approved among the native Americans. The name, Indian tobacco, given to *Lobelia inflata*, L. (the emetic-weed of Cutler, *l. c.*, p. 484; who "first attracted to it the attention of the profession "), by the whites, is in some connections confusing, and might well be displaced by wild tobacco, which is also in popular use.

[3] *Œnothera biennis*, L. (Johnson's Gerard, p. 475),— known to Europeans, according to Linnæus (Sp. Pl., p. 493), as early as 1614; but first described and figured by Prosper Alpinus, in his posthumous *De Pl. Exoticis*, p. 325, t. 324, *cit.* L. Johnson says that Parkinson gave it the English name of tree-primrose, which it still keeps. It is "vulgarly known by the name of scabish (a corruption, probably of scabious)" in the country.— *Bigel. Fl. Bost., in loco.* Josselyn describes the plant in his Voyages, p. 78.

Maiden Hair, or *Cappellus veneris verus*, which ordinarily is half a Yard in height. The *Apothecaries* for
fhame now will fubftitute *Wall-Rue* no more for *Maiden
Hair*, fince it grows in abundance in *New-England*, from
whence they may have good ftore.[1]

Pirola, Two kinds. See the Figures, both of them
excellent Wound Herbs.[2]

Homer's Molley.[3]

[56] *Lyfimachus* or *Loofe Strife*, it grows in dry
grounds in the open Sun four foot high, Flowers from
the middle of the Plant to the top, the Flowers purple,
ftanding upon a fmall fheath or cod, which when it is
ripe breaks and puts forth a white filken doun, the ftalk
is red, and as big as ones Finger.[4]

Marygold of Peru, of which there are two kinds, one
bearing black feeds, the other black and white ftreak'd,
this beareth the faireft flowers, commonly but one upon
the very top of the ftalk.[5]

---

[1] *Adiantum pedatum*, L.—The European *A. Capillus veneris*, L., long used
as a pectoral (the *sirop de capillaire* of French shops being made of it), is, according to Messrs. Wood and Bache (Dispens., p. 1290), "feebler" than our
species, which Josselyn recommends.

[2] See pp. 67, 68.

[3] Johnson's Gerard, p. 183: which is perhaps *Allium magicum*, L.; for which
our *A. tricoccum*, Ait., may have been mistaken. — See also p. 54 of this; note.

[4] *Epilobium angustifolium*, L. (rosebay willow-herbe of Gerard by Johnson);
which last figures it at p. 477: common to Europe and America; but some
botanists have, like Josselyn, reckoned the American plant "proper to the
country."

Helianthus, L. (Gerard, p. 751), a genus peculiar to America; called
"American marygold" in the Voyages (p. 59), where it is set down among the
more striking of our New-England flowers. At p. 82 of this book, the author
gives a cut of the "marygold of America," which he describes. It is probably

Treacle-Berries. See before *Salomons Seal.*
Oak of Hierufalem. See before.
Oak of Cappadocca. See before.
Earth-Nuts, differing much from thofe in *England*, one
fort of them bears a moft beautiful Flower.[1]

For the Scurvy and Dropfie.

Sea-Tears, they grow upon the Sea banks in abundance, they are good for the Scurvy and Dropfie, boiled
and eaten as a Sallade, and the broth drunk with it.[2]

Indian Beans, better for Phyfick ufe than other Beans.

Indian Beans, falfly called *French beans*, are better for
Phyfick and Chyrurgery [57] than our Garden Beans.
Probatum eft :[3]

---

the second one above mentioned, and perhaps *H. strumosus*, L., Gray. The
other kind, with "black seeds," was probably *H. divaricatus*, L.

[1] See p. 47. The earth-nuts of Gerard (p. 1064) are species of *Bulbocastanum*
of authors.

[2] Not clear to me. But, taking the alleged virtues and the station into account, our author may mean here the rather striking American sea-rocket (*Cakile
Americana*, Nutt.); which, it is likely, occurred to him. Spurge-time (p. 43)
also grows on "sea-banks."

[3] "French beans; or, rather, American beans. The herbalists call them
kidney-beans, from their shape and effects; for they strengthen the kidneys.
They are variegated much, — some being bigger, a great deal, than others; some
white, black, red, yellow, blue, spotted : besides your *Bonivis*, and *Calavances*,
and the kidney-bean that is proper to Ronoake. But these are brought into the
country : the other are natural to the climate." — *Josselyn's Voyages*, p. 73-4. R.
Williams (Key, *l. c.*, p. 208) gives *manusquussedash* as the Indian word for beans.
Cornuti (whose book, indeed, is not confined to Canadian plants; though, on
the other hand, he was sometimes ill informed of the true locality of his specimens; as in the case of *Asclepias Cornuti*, Decsne, which he published as *A.
Syriaca*) figures and describes, at pp. 184-5, *Phaseolus multiflorus*, L.; and this

Squaſhes, but more truly *Squonterſquaſhes*, a kind of
Mellon, or rather Gourd, for they oftentimes degenerate
into Gourds; ſome of theſe are green, ſome yellow,
ſome longiſh like a Gourd, others round like an Apple,
all of them pleaſant food boyled and buttered, and ſea-
ſon'd with Spice; but the yellow *Squaſh* called an Apple
Squaſh, becauſe like an Apple, and about the bigneſs of
a Pome-water is the beſt kind;[1] they are much eaten by
the *Indians* and the *Engliſh*, yet they breed the ſmall
white Worms (which Phyſitians call *Aſcarides*,) in the
long Gut that vex the Fundament with a perpetual itch-
ing, and a deſire to go to ſtool.

Water-Mellon, it is a large Fruit, but nothing near ſo
big as a Pompion, colour, ſmoother, and of a ſad Graſs
green rounder or more rightly *Sap-green* ; with ſome
yellowneſs admixt when ripe; the ſeeds are black, the
fleſh or pulpe exceeding juicy.[2]

---

may possibly have been raised from seeds procured by French missionaries from
the Canadian savages : but *P. vulgaris*, L., our well-known bush-bean, is doubtless what Josselyn has mainly in view, as cultivated by the native Americans.

[1] "*Askutasquash*, — their vine-apples, — which the English, from them, call
squashes : about the bigness of apples of several colours." — *R. Williams, Key,
&c., l. c.*, p. 222. "In summer, when their corn is spent, *isquotersquashes* is their
best bread : a fruit much like a pumpion." — *Wood, New-Eng. Prospect*, part 2,
chap. vi. The late Dr. T. W. Harris made the ill-understood edible gourds a
special object of study, and devoted particular attention to the ascertaining of the
kinds cultivated by the American savages; but his papers have not as yet seen
the light. The warted squash (*Cucurbita verrucosa*, L.) and the orange-gourd
(*C. aurantium*, Willd.) — the fruit of which last is of the size and color of an
orange, and "more tender than the common pompion" (Loudon, Encycl. Pl.) —
are perhaps, in part, intended by our author.

[2] "Pompions and water-mellons, too, they have good store," says our author
(Voyages, p. 130); and again, at p. 74 of the same, "The water-melon is proper

For heat and thirſt in Feavers.

It is often given to thoſe ſick of Feavers, and other hot Diſeaſes with good ſucceſs.

[58] *New-England Dayſie,* or *Primroſe,* is the ſecond kind of *Navel Wort* in *Johnſon* upon *Gerard*; it flowers in *May,* and grows amongſt Moſs upon hilly Grounds and Rocks that are ſhady.[1]

---

to the countrie. The fleſh of it is of a fleſh-colour; a rare cooler of feavers, and excellent against the stone." The water-melon (*Cucurbita citrullus,* L.) is " the only medicine the common people use in ardent fevers," in Egypt (Loudon, *l. c.*). *Cucurbita pepo,* L. (Gr. πέπων; Low Dutch, *pepoen, pompoen;* Fr., *pompone*), is our English pompion, or pumpkin. At p. 91, Josselyn speaks of pompions "proper to the country." Compare Gerard's chapter " of melons, or pompions" (Johnson's Gerard, p. 918), where are two Virginian sorts; and see "the ancient New-England standing dish," at p. 91 of this book. The evidence appears to be sufficient, that our savages had in cultivation, together with their corn and tobacco, — and, like these, derived originally from tropical regions, — several sorts of what we call squashes, some kinds of pompion, and also water-melons; and, Graves's letter (New-England Plantation, *l. c.,* p. 124) adds, musk-melons. See further, especially, Champlain (Voy. de la Nouv. France, *passim*) and L'Escarbot (Hist. de la Nouv. France, vol. ii. p. 836). Mr. A. De Candolle (Geogr. Bot., vol. ii. pp. 899, 904) disputes the American origin of the edible gourds, but does not appear to have examined all the early authorities for their cultivation by the savages before the settlement of this country. Such cultivation appears to be made out, and to indicate that these vegetables have probably been known, from very remote antiquity, in the warmer parts of America. But this does not touch the difficult question of origin; and it may still appear that the gourds are equally ancient in Europe, and derived, both here and there, from Asia (De Cand., *l. c.*); such derivation being explainable, in the case of America, by old migrations from Asia through Polynesia. — *Pickering, Races of Man,* chap. 17.

[1] Johnson's Gerard, p. 528; where the same plant is also called "jagged or rose penniwoort," and is probably what our author intends at p. 43 of this. It was no doubt our pretty *Saxifraga Virginiensis,* Michx., which Josselyn had in view. In his Voyages, p. 80, he assigns to it the medicinal virtues which Gerard attributes to the great navel-wort, or wall-pennywort (*Cotyledon umbilicus,* Huds.).

For Burns and Scalds.

It is very good for Burns and Scalds.

An Acharistion, or Medicine deserving thanks.

An *Indian* whose Thumb was .swell'd, and very much inflamed, and full of pain, increasing and creeping along to the wrist, with little black spots under the Thumb against the Nail; I Cured it with this *Umbellicus veneris* Root and all, the Yolk of an Egg, and Wheat flower, *f. Cata-plasme.*

Briony of Peru, (we call it though it grown hear) or rather *Scammony*; some take it for *Mechoacan*: The green Juice is absolutely Poyson; yet the Root when dry may safely be given to strong Bodies.[1]

Red and *Black Currence.* See before.

Wild Damask Roses, single, but very large and sweet, but stiptick.[2]

Sweet Fern,[3] the Roots run one within another like a

---

[1] *Convolvulus sepium,* L. (great bind-weed) is exceedingly like to *C. Scammonia,* L., the inspissated juice of which is the officinal scammony; and is common to Europe and North America. Gerard's bryony of Peru (p. 872-3), to which Josselyn refers, is, whatever it be, not found here. Compare Cutler's remarks on *C. sepium* (Account of Veg., &c., *l. c.,* p. 416). *Mechoacan,* "called . . . Indian briony, or briony, or scammony of America," from the Caribbee Islands, &c., is described in Hughes, Amer. Physitian (1672), p. 94; and see Wood and Bache, Dispens., p. 424, note.

[2] *Rosa Carolina,* L. (Carolina rose), probably. — See Cutler's observations, *l. c.,* p. 451. Higginson also notices "single damaske roses, verie sweete." — *New-Eng. Plantation, l. c.,* p. 119. Our Carolina rose is said to be common in English shrubberies.

[3] See also Voyages, p. 72. Our author is the earliest authority that I have met with for this name; and his plant, which is placed among those "proper to

Net, being very long and spreading abroad under the
upper cruft of [59] the Earth, fweet in tafte, but withal
aftringent, much hunted after by our Swine: The *Scotch-
men* that are in *New-England* have told me that it grows
in *Scotland*.

For Fluxes.

The People boyl the tender tops in *Moloſſes* Beer, and in
Poſſets for Fluxes, for which it is excellent.

Sarſaparilia, a Plant not yet fufficiently known by the
Engliſh : Some fay it is a kind of *Bind Weed*; we have,
in *New-England* two Plants, that go under the name of
Sarſaparilia: the one not above a foot in height without
Thorns, the other having the fame Leaf, but is a fhrub as
high as a *Gooſe Berry Buſh*, and full of fharp Thorns;
this I efteem as the right, by the fhape and favour of the
Roots, but rather by the effects anfwerable to that we
have from other parts of the World; It groweth upon
dry Sandy banks by the Sea fide, and upon the banks of
Rivers, fo far as the Salt water flowes ; and within Land
up in the Country, as fome have reported.[1]

---

the country," may very well be what has long been called sweet-fern in New
England, — *Comptonia asplenifolia* (L.) Ait.; still used in "molasses beer,"
and medicinal in the way mentioned. — *Emerson, Trees and Shrubs of Mass.*,
p. 226.

[1] See Josselyn's Voyages, p. 77. The first of the two plants which the author
mentions here is probably *Aralia nudicaulis*, L. (wild sarsaparilla); and the
other, *A. hispida*, Michx. The last. which is what is spoken of in the Voyages,
has been recommended for medicinal properties by Prof. Peck. — *Wood and
Bache, Dispens.*, p. 116.

Bill Berries, two kinds, Black and Sky Coloured, which is more frequent.[1]

[60] *To cool the heat of Feavers, and quench Thirſt.*

They are very good to allay the burning heat of Feavers, and hot Agues, either in Syrup or Conſerve.

A moſt excellent Summer Diſh.

They uſually eat of them put into a Baſon, with Milk, and ſweetned a little more with Sugar and Spice, or for cold Stomachs, in Sack. The *Indians* dry them in the Sun, and ſell them to the *Engliſh* by the *Buſhell,* who make uſe of them inſtead of Currence, putting of them into Puddens, both boyled and baked, and into Water Gruel.

Knot Berry, or *Clowde Berry,* ſeldom ripe.[2]

---

[1] "*Attitaash* (whortleberries), of which there are divers sorts; sweet, like currants; some opening, some of a binding nature. *Sautaash* are these currants dried by the natives, and so preserved all the year; which they beat to powder, and mingle it with their parched meal, and make a delicate dish which they call *sautauthig,* which is as sweet to them as plum or spice cake to the English." — *R. Williams, Key, &c., l. c.,* p. 221. The fruitful and wholesome American whortleberries, or bilberries, were, it is likely, a very pleasant discovery to our forefathers. It was, no doubt, those species that we call blueberries which they made most of, and particularly the low blueberry (*Vaccinium Pennsylvanicum,* Lam.) and the swamp-blueberry (*V. corymbosum,* L.). From these the common black whortleberry (*Gaylussacia resinosa,* Torr. and Gray) differs no less in quality than in structure. *Sa'té* (compare *sautaash,* above), in Rasles Dict. of the Abnaki Language, *l. c.,* p. 450, is rendered "*frais, sans etre secs; lorsq'ils s't secs, sikisa'tar.*"

[2] The cloud-berry — *Rubus chamœmorus,* L. (Gerard, p. 1420) — is found in some parts of the subalpine region of the White Mountains; and Mr. Oakes detected it at Lubec, on the coast of Maine. It is common to both continents;

Sumach, differing from all that I did ever fee in the Herbalifts; our *Englifh* Cattle devour it moft abominably, leaving neither Leaf nor Branch, yet it fprouts again next Spring.[1]

For Colds.

The *Englifh* ufe to boyl it in Beer, and drink it for Colds; and fo do the *Indians,* from whom the *Englifh* had the Medicine.

Wild Cherry, they grow in clufters like [61] Grapes, of the fame bignefs, blackifh, red when ripe, and of a harfh tafte.[2]

For Fluxes.

They are alfo good for Fluxes.

Tranfplanted and manured, they grow exceeding fair.

---

and perhaps, therefore, as our author gives his cloud-berry a place in this division of his book, he may have meant something else.

[1] *Rhus,* L.; the species differing, as our author repeats in his Voyages (p. 71), "from all the kinds set down in our English herbals." Wood (N. Eng. Prospect, chap. v.) calls it "the dear shumach." Josselyn's account of the virtues of our species, here, and especially in the Voyages (*l. c.*), agrees so well with what Gerard says of the properties of the European tanner's sumach (*R. coriaria,* L.), that the latter may very likely have, in part, suggested the former. But see Cutler, *l. c.,* p. 427.

[2] "The cherry-trees yield great store of cherries, which grow on clusters like grapes. They be much smaller than our English cherry; nothing near so good, if they be not fully ripe. They so furr the mouth, that the tongue will cleave to the roof, and the throat wax hoarse with swallowing those red bullies (as I may call them); being little better in taste" (that is, than bullaces). "English ordering may bring them to an English cherry; but they are as wild as the Indians." — *New-England's Prospect,* chap. v. The choke-cherry (*Cerasus Virginiana* (L.) DC.) and the wild cherry (*C. serotina* (Ehrh.) DC.) are meant.

Board Pine, is a very large Tree two or three Fadom about.[1]

For Wounds.

It yields a very foveraign Turpentine for the Curing of defperate Wounds.

For Stabbs.

The *Indians* make ufe of the *Mofs* boiled in Spring Water, for Stabbs, pouring in the Liquor, and applying the boiled Mofs well ftamp'd or beaten betwixt two ftones.

For Burning and Scalding.

And for Burning and Scalding, they firft take out the fire with a ftrong decoction of Alder Bark, then they lay upon it a Playfter of the bark of *Board Pine* firft boyled tender, and beat to a Playfter betwixt two ftones.

To take Fire out of a Burn.

One *Chriftopher Luxe*, a Fifher-man, having burnt his Knee Pan, was healed [62] again by an *Indian Webb*, or Wife, (for fo they call thofe Women that have Husbands;) She firft made a ftrong decoction of Alder bark, with which fhe took out the Fire by Imbrocation, or letting of

---

[1] *Pinus Strobus*, L. (white pine). "Of the body the English make large canows of 20 foot long, and two foot and a half over; hollowing of them with an adds, and shaping of the outside like a boat."— *Josselyn's Voyages*, p. 64; where is more concerning the use of this tree in medicine. "I have seen," says Wood, "of these stately, high-grown trees, ten miles together, close by the river-side; from whence, by shipping, they might be conveyed to any desired port."— *New-Eng. Prospect*, chap. v.

it drop upon the Sore, which would fmoak notably with it; then fhe Playftered it with the Bark of *Board Pine*, or *Hemlock Tree*, boyled foft and ftampt betwixt two ftones, till it was as thin as brown Paper, and of the fame Colour, fhe annointed the Playfter with *Soyles Oyl*, and the Sore likewife, then fhe laid it on warm, and fometimes fhe made ufe of the bark of the *Larch Tree*.

To eat out proud Flefh in a Sore.

And to eat out the proud Flefh, they take a kind of *Earth Nut* boyled and ftamped, and laft of all, they apply to the Sore the Roots of *Water Lillies* boiled and ftamped betwixt two ftones, to a Playfter.

For Stitches.

The *Firr Tree*, or *Pitch Tree*,[1] the Tar that is made of all forts of *Pitch Wood* is an excellent thing to take away thofe defperate Stitches of the Sides, which perpetually afflicteth thofe poor People that are [63] ftricken with the *Plague of the Back.*

---

[1] *Abies balsamea* (L.) Marsh. (balsam-fir). "The firr-tree is a large tree, too; but seldom so big as the pine. The bark is smooth, with knobs, or blisters, in which lyeth clear liquid turpentine, — very good to be put into salves and oynt-ments. The leaves, or cones, boiled in beer, are good for the scurvie. The young buds are excellent to put into epithemes for warts and corns. The rosen is altogether as good as frankincense. . . . The knots of this tree and fat-pine are used by the English instead of candles; and it will burn a long time: but it makes the people pale" (Josselyn's Voyages, p. 66); besides being, as Wood says (*l. c.*, speaking of the pine), "something sluttish." But Higginson says they "are very usefull in a house, and . . . burne as cleere as a torch." — *New-Eng. Plantation, l. c.*, p. 122.

Note, You muſt make a large Toaſt, or Cake ſlit and dip it in the Tar, and bind it warm to the Side.

The moſt common Diſeaſes in New England.

The *Black Pox,* the *Spotted Feaver,* the *Griping of the Guts,* the *Dropſie,* and the *Sciatica,* are the killing Diſeaſes in *New-England.*

The *Larch Tree,* which is the only Tree of all the Pines, that ſheds his Leaves before Winter; The other remaining Green all the Year: This is the Tree from which we gather that uſeful purging.excrenſe, *Agarick.*[1]

For Wounds and Cuts.

The Leaves and Gum are both very good to heal Wounds and Cuts.

For Wounds with Bruiſes.

I cured once a deſperate Bruiſe with a Cut upon the Knee Pan, with an Ungent made with the Leaves of the Larch Tree, and Hogs Greaſe, but the Gum is beſt.

Spruce is a goodly Tree, of which they make Maſts for Ships, and Sail Yards: It is generally conceived by thoſe

---

[1] *Larix Americana,* Michx. (Larch; "*taccamahac.*" Cutler; *tamarack; hackmatack.*) "Groundsels, made of larch-tree, will never rot; and the longer it lyes, the harder it growes, that you may almost drive a nail into a bar of iron as easily as into that." — *Josselyn's Voyages,* p. 68. "The turpentine that issueth from the cones of the larch-tree (which comes nearest of any to the right turpentine) is singularly good to heal wounds, and to draw out the malice (or thorn, as Helmont phrases it) of any ach; rubbing the place therewith, and throwing upon it the powder of sage-leaves." — *Ibid.,* p. 66.

that have [64] skill in Building of Ships, that here is abſolutely the beſt Trees in the World, many of them being three Fathom about, and of great length.[1]

An Achariſton for the Scurvy.

The tops of Green *Spruce* Boughs boiled in *Bear*, and drunk, is aſſuredly one of the beſt Remedies for the Scurvy, reſtoring the Infected party in a ſhort time; they alſo make a Lotion of ſome of the decoction, adding Hony and Allum.

Hemlock Tree, a kind of *Spruce*, the bark of this Tree ſerves to dye Tawny; the Fiſhers Tan their Sails and Nets with it.[2]

---

[1] *Abies nigra*, Poir. (black or double spruce), and probably also *A. alba*, Michx. (white or single spruce). "At Pascataway there is now a spruce-tree, brought down to the water-side by our mass-men, of an incredible bigness, and so long that no skipper durst ever yet adventure to ship it; but there it lyes and rots." — *Josselyn's Voyages*, p. 67.

[2] *Abies Canadensis* (L.), Michx. (hemlock spruce). Beside the coniferous trees here set down, our author mentions in his Voyages (p. 67) "the white cedar, . . . a stately tree, and is taken by some to be tamarisk." This, which is probably our white cedar (*Cupressus thyoides*, L.), he says "the English saw into boards to floor their rooms; for which purpose it is excellent, long-lasting, and wears very smooth and white. Likewise they make shingles to cover their houses with, instead of tyle. It will never warp." Wood (New-Eng. Prospect, chap. v.) makes mention of a "cedar-tree, . . . a tree of no great growth; not bearing above a foot and a half, at the most; neither is it very high. . . . This wood is more desired for ornament than substance; being of colour red and white, like eugh; smelling as sweet as juniper. It is commonly used for ceiling of houses, and making of chests, boxes, and staves." This seems likely to have been the American *Arbor vitæ* (*Thya occidentalis*, L.); also called white-cedar. — Compare Emerson, Trees and Shrubs of Mass., pp. 96, 100. For mention of the juniper, see *ante*, p. 49.

To break Sore or Swelling.

The *Indians* break and heal their Swellings and Sores with it, boyling the inner Bark of young *Hemlock* very well, then knocking of it betwixt two ftones to a Playfter, and annointing or foaking it in Soyls Oyl, they apply it to the Sore: It will break a Sore Swelling fpeedily.

One Berry, Herba Paris, or *True Love.*[1]
Saffafras, or *Ague Tree.*[2]

[65] *For heat in Feavers.*

The Chips of the Root boyled in Beer is excellent to allay the hot rage of Feavers, being drunk.

For Bruifes and dry Blowes.

The Leaves of the fame Tree are very good made into an Oyntment, for Bruifes and dry Blows. The Bark of the Root we ufe inftead of Cinamon; and it is Sold at the *Barbadoes* for two Shillings the Pound.

And why may not this be the Bark the Jefuits Powder was made of, that was fo Famous not long fince in *England,* for Agues?

Cran Berry, or *Bear Berry,* becaufe Bears ufe much to

---

[1] See p. 81; and *ante,* p. 54.
[2] *Sassafras officinale.* Nees. " This tree growes not beyond Black Point, eaftward."— *Josselyn's Voyages,* p. 68. Michaux (Sylva, vol. ii. p. 144) says, " The neighbourhood of Portsmouth . . . may be assumed as one of the extreme points at which it is found towards the north-eaft;" but, according to Mr. Emerson (Trees and Shrubs of Mass., p. 322), it is "found as far north as Canada," though . . . " there a small tree."

feed upon them, is a fmall trayling Plant that grows in Salt Marfhes that are over-grown with Mofs; the tender Branches (which are reddifh) run out in great length, lying flat on the ground, where at diftances, they take Root, over-fpreading fometimes half a fcore Acres, fometimes in fmall patches of about a Rood or the like; the Leaves are like Box, but greener, thick and gliftering; the Bloffoms are very like the Flowers of [66] our *Englifh Night Shade*, after which fucceed the Berries, hanging by long fmall foot ftalks, no bigger than a hair; at firft they are of a pale yellow Colour, afterwards red, and as big as a Cherry; fome perfectly round, others Oval, all of them hollow, of a fower aftringent tafte; they are ripe in *Auguft* and *September*.[1]

For the Scurvy.

They are excellent againft the Scurvy.

---

[1] *Vaccinium macrocarpum*, Ait. Our author feems not to have known the European cranberry (*V. oxycoccus*, L., the marish-wortes, or fenne-berries, of Gerard, p. 1419); which is also found in our cold bogs, especially upon mountains. This is called by Sir W. J. Hooker (Br. Fl., vol. i. p. 178), "far superior to the foreign *V. macrocarpon;*" but, from Gerard's account, it should appear that it was formerly much less thought of in England than was ours (according to Josselyn) here, by both Indians and English. Linnæus speaks of the European fruit in much the same way, in 1737, in his Flora of Lapland, where he says, "*Baccæ hæ a Lapponibus in usum cibarium non vocantur, nec facile ab aliis nationibus, cum nimis acidæ sint*" (Fl. Lapp., p. 145): but corrects this in a paper on the esculent plants of Sweden, in 1752; asking, not without animation, "*Harum vero cum saccharo præparata gelatina, quid in mensis nostris jucundius?*" (Amæn. Acad., t. iii. p. 86.) Our American cranberry was probably the "*sasemineash* — another sharp, cooling fruit, growing in fresh waters all the winter; excellent in conserve against fevers"—of R. Williams, Key, *l. c.*, p. 221.—Compare *Masimin*, rendered [*fruits*] "*rouges petits.*"—*Rasles' Dict., Abnaki, l. c.*, p. 460.

For the heat in Feavers.

They are alfo good to allay the fervour of hot Difeafes. The *Indians* and *Englifh* ufe them much, boyling them ,with Sugar for Sauce to eat with their Meat; and it is a delicate Sauce, efpecially for roafted Mutton: Some make Tarts with them as with Goofe Berries.

Vine, much differing in the Fruit, all of them very flefhy, fome reafonably pleafant; others have a tafte of Gun Powder, and thefe grow in Swamps, and low wet Grounds.[1]

---

[67] 3. *Of fuch Plants as are proper to the Country, and have no Name.*

(I.)

P*Irola,* or *Winter Green,* that kind which grows with us in *England* is common in *New-England,*[2] but

---

[1] Wood says the "vines afford great store of grapes, which are very big, both for the grape and cluster; sweet and good. These be of two sorts, — red and. white. There is likewise a smaller kind of grape which groweth in the islands" (that is, of Massachusetts Bay). "which is sooner ripe, and more delectable; so that there is no known reason why as good wine may not be made in those parts, as well as Bordeaux in France; being under the same degree." — *New-Eng. Prospect,* chap. v. "Vines," says Mr. Graves (in New-Eng. Plantation, Hist. Coll., vol. i. p. 124) "doe grow here. plentifully laden with the biggest grapes that ever I saw. Some I have seene foure inches about." — "Our Governour," adds Higginson, "hath already planted a vineyard, with great hope of encrease." — *New-England's Plantation. l. c.,* p. 119. *Vitis Labrusca,* L. (fox-grape), — for some principal varieties of which, see Emerson, *l. c.,* p. 468, — furnished, probably, most of the sorts known favorably to the first settlers; but *V. æstivalis,* Michx. (summer grape), also occurs on our seaboard.

[2] *Pyrola,* L., emend. (Gerard, p. 408). All but one of our species are common also to Europe.

P

there is another plant which I judge to be a kind of *Pirola*, and proper to this Country, a very beautiful Plant; The shape of the Leaf and the just bignefs of it you may fee in the Figure. ♠

The Leaf of the Plant judged to be a kind of Pirola.

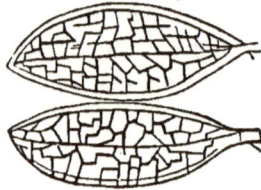

The Ground whereof is a Sap Green, embroydered (as it were) with many pale yellow Ribs, the whole Plant in fhape is [68] like *Semper vivum*, but far lefs, being not above a handful high, with one flender ftalk, adorned with fmall pale yellow Flowers like the other *Pirola*. It groweth not every where, but in fome certain fmall fpots overgrown with Mofs, clofe by fwamps and fhady; they are green both Summer and Winter.[1]

For Wounds.

They are excellent Wound Herbs, but this I judge to be the better by far. *Probatum eft.*

---

[1] *Goodyera pubescens* (Willd.), R. Br., is plainly meant by the author; and the common name of the plant — rattlesnake plantain — still preferves the memory of its supposed virtues as a wound-herb. It feems, by the next page, that Joffelyn tried to carry living specimens to England; but they "perished at sea." The putting this among the *Pyrolæ* (as if by some confufion of *Goodyera* with *Chimophila maculata*) was a bad mistake.

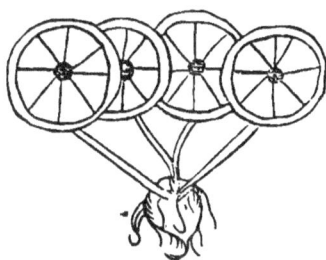

2.

This Plant was brought to me by a neighbour, who (wandering in the Woods to find out his ſtrayed Cattle,) loſt himſelf [69] for two Dayes, being as he gheſſed eight or ten Miles from the Sea-ſide. The Root was pretty thick and black, having a number of ſmall black ſtrings growing from it, the ſtalks of the Leaves about a handful long, the Leaves were round and as big as a Silver five Shilling piece, of a ſap or dark green Colour, with a line or ribb as black as Jeat round the Circumference, from whence came black lines or ribs at equal diſtance, all of them meeting in a black ſpot in the Center.[1]

---

[1] See p. 55; where the author refers to his figures of two kinds of "*Pyrola*," of which this must be one. The Voyages (p. 202) also make mention of an adventure of a neighbor of Joſselyn's, who, "rashly wandering out after some ſtray'd cattle, lost his way; and coming, as we conceived by his Relation, near to the head-ſpring of some of the branches of Black-Point River or Saco River, light into a tract of land, for God knows how many miles, full of delfes and dingles and dangerous precipices, rocks, and inextricable difficulties, which did juſtly daunt, yea, quite deter him from endeavouring to pass any further." And this account may quite possibly relate to the same occasion of our author's getting acquainted with his "elegant plant." Plukenet (Amalth., p. 94; Phytogr., tab. 287, f. 5) mistakenly refers Josselyn's "sufficiently unhappy figure" to his *Filix Hemionitis dicta Maderensis;* which is *Adiantum reniforme,* L.

If I had ſtaid longer in the Country, I ſhould have pur-
poſely made a Journey into thoſe Parts where it was
gathered, to diſcover if poſſible, the Stalk and Flower;
but now I ſhall refer it to thoſe that are younger, and
better able to undergo the pains and trouble of finding it
out; for I underſtood by the Natives, that it is not common, that is, every where to be found, no more then the
embroydered *Pirola*, which alſo is a moſt elegant Plant,
and which I did endeavour to bring over, but it periſhed at
Sea.

For Wounds.

Clownes all heal, of *New-England,* is another Wound
Herb not Inferiour to [70] ours, but rather beyond it:
Some of our *Engliſh* practitioners take it for *Vervene,* and
uſe it for the ſame, wherein they are groſly miſtaken.

The Leaf is like a Nettle Leaf, but narrower and
longer; the ſtalk about the bigneſs of a Nettle ſtalk,
Champhered and hollow, and of a dusky red Colour;
the Flowers are blew, ſmall, and many, growing in ſpoky
tufts at the top, and are not hooded, but having only four
round Leaves, after which followeth an infinite of ſmall
longiſh light brown Seed; the Roots are knotty and
matted together with an infinite number of ſmall white
ſtrings; the whole Plant is commonly two Cubits high,
bitter in taſte, with a Roſenic favour.[1]

---

1 "There is a plant, likewiſe, — called, for want of a name, clowne's wound-
wort, by the Engliſh; though it be not the ſame, — that will heal a green wound
in 24 hours, if a wiſe man have the ordering of it." — *Voyages,* p. 60. *Verbena*

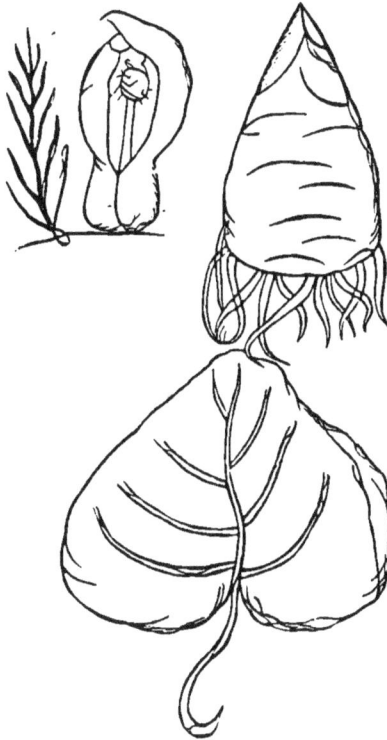

(3.)

This Plant is one of the firſt that ſprings up after White

---

hastata. L. (blue vervain), is perhaps, notwithstanding the author's disclaimer, what he had in view. This is certainly different from the common, once officinal, vervain of Europe (*V. officinalis*, L.), — on the virtues of which, as a wound-herb. see Gerard, p. 718; but yet more so from true clown's all-heal (Gerard, p. 1005), which is *Stachys palustris*, L. As to other medicinal properties of our vervains, compare Cutler, *l. c.*, p. 405, — where they are said to have been used by the surgeons of our army in the Revolutionary War, — and Wood and Bache, Dispens., p. 1403.

Hellibore, in the like wet and black grounds, commonly by *Hellibore,* with a fheath or Hood like Dragons, but the peftle is of another fhape, that is, having a round Purple Ball on the top of it, befet (as it were) with Burs; the hood fhoots forth immediately from the Root, before any Leaf appears, having a Green [72] fprig growing faft by it, like the fmaller *Horfe Tayl,* about the latter end of *April* the Hood and Sprig wither away, and there comes forth in the room a Bud, like the Bud of the *Walnut Tree,* but bigger; the top of it is of a pale Green Colour, covered with brown skins like an Onion, white underneath the Leaves, which fpread in time out of the Bud, grow from the root with a ftalk a Foot long, and are as big as the great *Bur Dock* Leaves, and of the colour; the Roots are many, and of the bignefs of the fteel of a Tobacco Pipe, and very white; the whole Plant fents as ftrong as a Fox; it continues till *Auguft.*[1]

[74] (4.)

This Plant the *Humming Bird* feedeth upon, it groweth likewife in wet grounds, and is not at its full growth till

---

[1] *Symplocarpus fœtidus* (L.) Salisb. (skunk-cabbage). Our author's appears to be the first figure and account of this curious plant, which he rightly places among such "as are proper to the country, and have no name." Cutler's description, in 1785 (Account of Indig. Veg., *l. c.,* pp. 407–9), — which is followed by the remark, that "the fructification so essentially differs from all the genera of this order, it must undoubtedly be considered as a new genus," — was the next contribution of importance, and so continued till Dr. Bigelow's elaborate history; — *Amer. Med. Bot.,* vol. ii. p. 41, pl. xxiv. Josselyn's "sprig" of a horse-tail might perhaps be added to his *Filices,* at p. 47, note 2, 3.

[73] *A Branch of the Humming Bird Tree.*

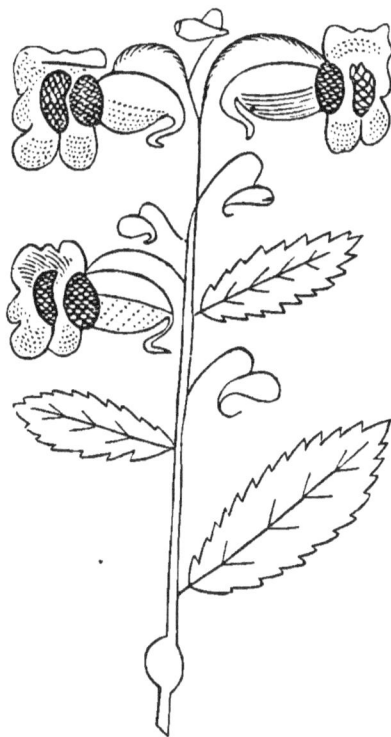

July, and then it is two Cubits high and better, the
Leaves are thin, and of a pale green Colour, some of them
as big as a Nettle Leaf, it spreads into many Branches,
knotty at the setting on, and of a purple Colour, and gar-
nished on the top with many hollow dangling Flowers of
a bright yellow Colour, speckled with a deeper yellow as

it were fhadowed, the Stalkes are as hollow as a Kix, and
fo are the Roots, which are tranfparent, very tender, and
full of a yellowifh juice.[1]

For Bruifes and Aches upon ftroaks.

The *Indians* make ufe of it for Aches, being bruifed
between two ftones, and laid tocold, but made (after the
Englifh manner) into an unguent with Hogs Greafe, there
is not a more foveraign remedy for bruifes of what kind
foever; and for Aches upon Stroaks.

In *Auguft*, 1670. in a Swamp amongft *Alders*, I found a
fort of Tree *Sow Thiftle*, the Stalks of fome two or three
Inches, [75] about, as hollow as a Kix and very brittle,
the Leaves were fmooth, and in fhape like *Sonchus lævis*,
i.e. *Hares Lettice*, but longer, fome about a Foot, thefe
grow at a diftance one from another, almoft to the top,
where it begins to put forth Flowers between the Leaves

---

[1] *Impatiens fulva*, Nutt. (touch-me-not; balsam). Wilson says this plant
" is the greatest favorite with the humming-bird of all our other flowers. In some
places where these plants abound, you may see at one time ten or twelve hum-
ming-birds darting about, and fighting with and pursuing each other." —*Amer.
Ornithol., by Brewer*, p. 120. As to Josselyn's note on its use in medicine by the
Indians, compare Wood and Bache, Disp., p. 1345. A kix, or kex, or kexy, —
used in the expression, " hollow as a kix," — is a provincialism, in various parts
of England, for hemlock; " the dry, hollow stocks of hemlock " (whence Webster's
query, — Fr., *cigue*; Lat. *cicuta*); and also of cow-parsley, according to Holloway
(Dict. of Provincialisms): that is to say, secondarily, any hollow-stemmed plant
like hemlock. Gerard's figure of *Impatiens noli tangere*, L., the European balsam, — of which the earlier botanists considered our species to be varieties, — is
so poor, and the plant so rare in Britain, that it is perhaps little wonder that our
author took the showy American balsam to be quite new.

and the Stalk, the top of the stalk runs out into a spike, beset about with Flowers like Sow Thistle, of a blew or azure colour: I brought home one of the Plants which was between twelve and thirteen Foot in length, I wondered at it the more for that so large and tall a Plant should grow from so small a Root, consisting of slender white strings little bigger than Bents, and not many of them, and none above a Finger long, spreading under the upper crust of the Earth; the whole Plant is full of Milk, and of a strong favour.[1]

[76] *The Plant when it springs up first.*

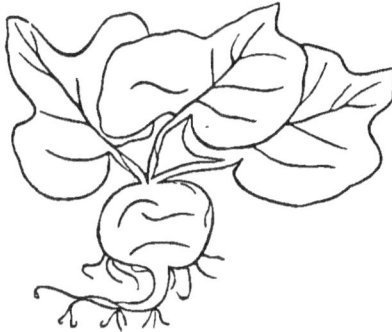

(5.)

This Plant I found in a gloomy dry Wood under an Oak, 1670. the 18*th* of *August*, afterwards I found it in

---

[1] *Mulgedium leucophæum*, DC. (Gray, Manual, p. 241). This fine plant is peculiar to America.

Q

[77] *The Figure of the Plant when it is at full growth.*

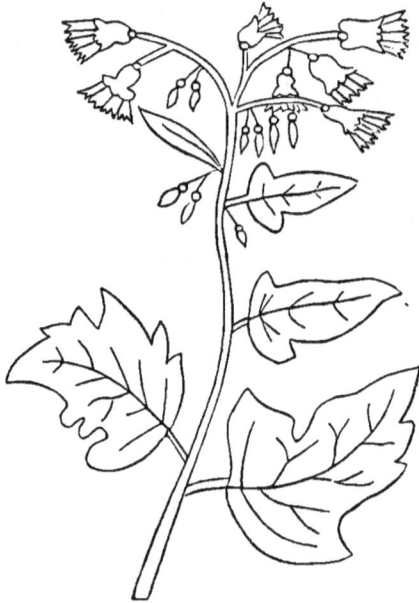

open Champain grounds, but yet fomewhat fcarce: The
Root is about the bignefs of a *French* Walnut, the Bark
thereof is brown, and rugged, within of a yellowifh
Colour, from whence arifeth a flender ftalk, no bigger
than an Oat ftraw, about two Cubits in height, fomewhat better than a handful above the Root fhooteth out
one Leaf of a Grafs Green colour, and an Inch or two
above that, another Leaf, and fo four or five at a greater
diftance one from another, till they come within a handful
of the top, where upon flender foot ftalks grow the Flow-

ers four or five, more or fewer, cluftering together in pale long green husks milk white, confifting of ten fmall Leaves, fnipt a little on the edges with purple hair threads in the midft; the whole Plant is of a brakifh taft: When it is at its full growth the ftalks are as red as Blood.[1]

[78]

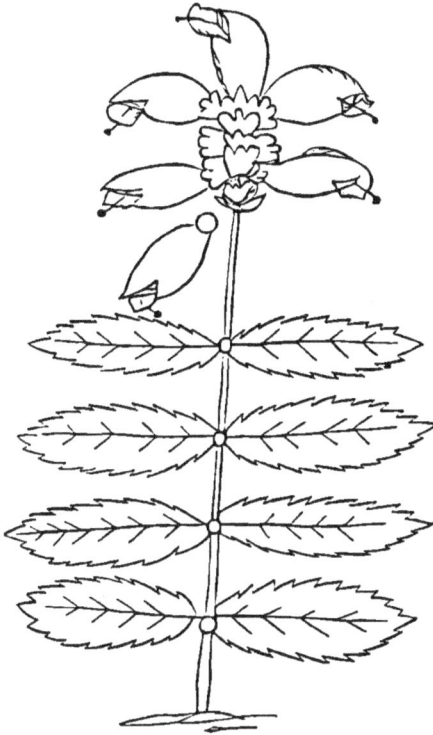

[1] *Nabalus albus* (L.) Hook. (Snake-weed) : the genus peculiar to America.

[79] (6.)

This Plant Flowers in *Auguſt*, and grows in wet Ground; it is about three or four foot in height, having a ſquare ſlender ſtalk, chamfered, hollow and tuff, the Leaves grow at certain diſtances one againſt another, of the colour of *Egrimony* Leaves ſharpe pointed, broadeſt in the midſt about an Inch and half, and three or four Inches in length, ſnipt about the edges like a Nettle Leaf, at the top of the Stalk for four or five Inches thick, ſet with pale green husks, out of which the Flowers grow, conſiſting of one Leaf, ſhaped like the head of a Serpent, opening at the top like a mouth, and hollow throughout, containing four crooked pointels, and on the top of every pointel a ſmall, gliſtering, green button, covered with a little white woolly matter, by which they are with the pointels faſtened cloſe together and ſhore up the tip of the upper chap, the crooked pointels are very ſtiff and hard, from the bottom of the husks, wherein the Flower ſtands, from the top of the Seed Veſſel ſhoots out a white thread which runs in at the bottom of the Flower, and ſo [80] out at the mouth; the whole Flower is milk white, the inſide of the chaps reddiſh, the Root I did not obſerve.[1]

---

[1] *Chelone glabra*, L. (snake-head). Plukenet quotes this figure under *Digitalis Verbesinæ foliis*, &c. (Amalth., p. 71; Mant., p. 64); which is referred by Linnæus to *Gerardia pedicularis*, L. Plukenet has himself figured our plant, and but little better than Josselyn, in Phytogr., t. 348, fig. 3. The genus is peculiar to America.

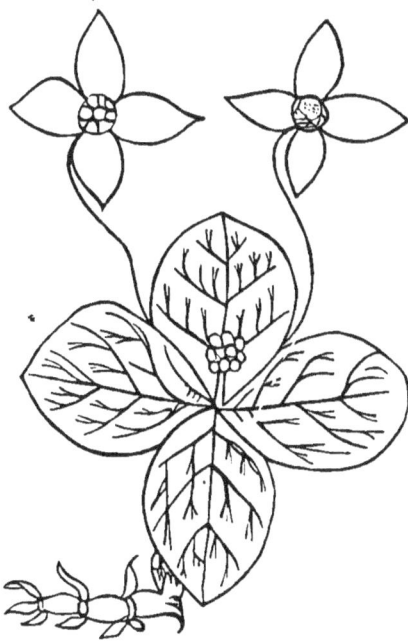

[81] (7.)

This Plant I take for a varigated Herb *Paris*, *True Love*
or *One Berry*, or rather *One Flower*, which is milk white,
and made up with four Leaves, with many black threads
in the middle, upon every thread grows a Berry (when
the Leaves of the Flower are fallen) as big as a white
peafe, of a light red colour when they are ripe, and cluster-
ing together in a round form as big as a Pullets Egg,
which at diſtance ſhews but as one Berry, very pleaſant
in taſte, and not unwholſome; the Root, Leaf, and

Flower differ not from our *Englifh* kind, and their time of blooming and ripening agree, and therefore doubtlefs a kind of *Herba Paris*.[1]

[82] *The fmall Sun Flower, or Marygold of America.*

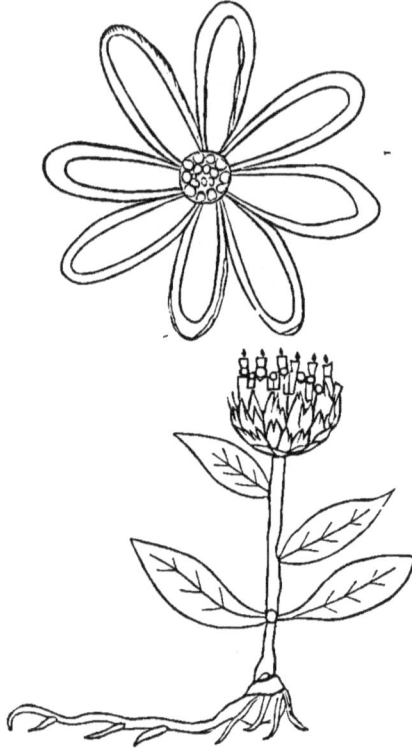

---

[1] Upon this figure, Plukenet founds his *Solanum quadrifolium Nov' Anglicanum, flore lacteo polycoccum* (Amalth., p. 195); clearly taking the plant, as Josselyn did, for "a kind of *Herba Paris*" (*Paris quadrifolia*, L.), which is *Solanum quadrifolium bacciferum* of Bauhin (Pin., p. 167, *cit.* L.). The plant is

[83]

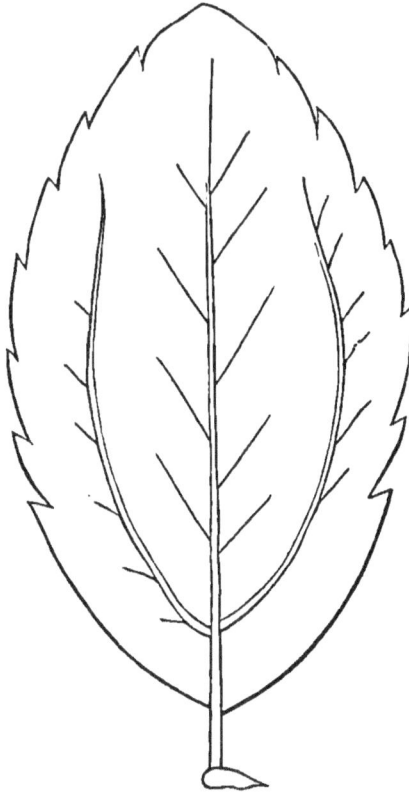

[84]   (8.)

This Plant is taken by our Simplifts to be a kind of

doubtless *Cornus Canadensis.* L. (dwarf-cornel; bunch-berry); and it certainly resembles the figure of *Herb Paris*, given by Gerard (p. 405), much more than that of *Cornus suecica*, L. (European dwarf-cornel, p. 1296), — a shrub ill understood by the old botanists.

Golden Rod, by others for *Sarazens Confound*. I judge it to be a kind of fmall *Sun Flower*, or *Marygold* of the *Weft Indies*; the Root is brown and flender, a foot and half in length, running a flope under the upper face of the Earth, with fome ftrings here and there, the ftalk as big as the fteal of a Tobacco pipe, full of pith, commonly brown-ifh, fometimes purple, three or four foot high, the Leaves grow at a diftance one againft another, rough, hard, green above, and gray underneath, flightly fnipt and the ribs appear moft on the back fide of the Leaf, the Flower is of a bright yellow, with little yellow cups in the midft, as in the *Marygold* of *Peru*, with black threads in them with yellow pointels, the Flower fpreads it felf abroad out of a cup made up of many green beards, not unlike a Thiftle; Within a handful of the top of the ftalk (when the Flower is fallen, growes an excrenfe or knob as big as a Walnut, which being broken yieldeth a kind of *Turpentine* or rather *Rofen*.[1]

What Cutchenele is.

The ftalk beneath and above the knob, covered with a multitude of fmall Bugs, about the bignefs of a great flea, which I prefume will make good *Cutchenele*, ordered as they fhould be before they come to have Wings: They make a perfect Scarlet Colour to Paint with, and durable.

---

[1] *Helianthus*, L., fp. (sun-flower); a genus peculiar to America. The species is perhaps *H. strumosus*, L. (Gray, Man., p. 218). — See p. [56] of this book; note.

4. *Of such Plants as have sprung up since the* English *Planted and kept Cattle in* New-England.[1]

C *Ouch Grass.*[2]
  Shepherds Purse.[3]
Dandelion.[4]
Groundsel.[5]
Sow Thistle.[6]

---

[1] The importance of this list has been already spoken of. Its value depends on its having been drawn up by a person of familiarity with some of the botanical writers of his day, as part of a botanical treatise; and the (in this case) not unfair presumption that the names cited are *meant* to be accurate. Mr. A. De Candolle (*Geogr. Botanique*, vol. ii. p. 746) appears to be unacquainted with any authority for the naturalized plants of the Northern States earlier than the first edition of the *Florula* of Dr. Bigelow, in 1814. The treatise of Cutler extends this limit to 1785; and that of Josselyn, so far as it goes, to 1672.

[2] Doubtful. Gerard's couch-grass, p. 23, appears to be *Holcus mollis*, L., — "the true couch-grass of sandy soils" in England; and English agricultural writers reckon yet other grasses of this name, beside the well-known *Triticum repens*, L.

[3] Gerard. p. 276. — *Capsella Bursa Pastoris* (L.), Moench. "Cornfields, and about barns." — *Cutler* (1785), *l. c.* Naturalized.

[4] Gerard, p. 290, — *Taraxacum Dens Leonis*, Desf.; looked, to our author, like a new-comer. Dr. Gray (Man., p. 239; and comp. Torr. and Gray, Fl., vol. ii. p. 494) regards it as "probably indigenous in the north," but only naturalized in other regions. "Grass land," — *Cutler* (1785), *l. c.*

[5] Gerard, p. 278, — *Senecio vulgaris*, L.; one of the *adventive* naturalized plants, as defined by Mr. De Candolle (*l. c.*, vol. ii. p. 688; and Gray, Man. Bot., pref., p. viii.), according to the evidence of Dr. Darlington (Fl. Cestr., p. 152), and Gray, *l. c.* It has long been a common weed in eastern New England.

[6] *Sonchus*, L. *S. oleraceus*, L., as understood by Linnæus, was no doubt intended: but this is now taken to include two species, both recognized in this country (Gray, *l. c.*, p. 241); between which there is no evidence to authorize a decision.

R

Wild Arrach.[1]

Night Shade, with the white Flower.[2]

Nettlesstinging, which was the first Plant taken notice of.[3]

Mallowes.[4]

[86] *Plaintain,* which the *Indians* call *Englissh-Mans Foot,* as though produced by their treading.[5]

---

[1] The *genera Chenopodium,* L., and *Atriplex,* L., were much confused in Josselyn's day; and his wild orach may belong to either. Gerard's wild orach is in part *Atriplex patula,* L. (p. 326); but the first species to which he gives this name (p. 325) is *Chenopodium polyspermum,* L. The latter is a rare, *adventive* member of our Flora (Gray, *l. c.,* p. 363); and the former is, according to Bigelow (Fl. Bost., ed. 3, p. 401), the well-known orach of our salt-marshes: but Dr. Gray now refers this (Man., p. 365) to the nearly allied *A. hastata,* L. This plant, in either case, is reckoned truly common to both continents. It is possible that Josselyn intended it.

[2] Garden nightshade (Gerard, p. 339); *Solanum nigrum,* L. "Common among rubbish," — *Cutler* (1785), *l. c.* Naturalized.

[3] Common stinging-nettle, or great nettle (Gerard, p. 706), — *Urtica dioica,* L.

[4] Field-mallow (Gerard, p. 930), *Malva sylvestris,* L., and wild dwarf-mallow (*ibid.*), *M. rotundifolia,* L., are the only sorts likely to have been in view. The latter was, I doubt not, intended; and the former, *adventive* only with us, may also have occurred at any period after the settlement.

[5] "It is but one sort, and that is broad-leaved plantain" (Josselyn's Voyages, p. 188). Broad-leaved plantain (Gerard, p. 419), — *Plantago major,* L.; one of the most anciently and widely known of plants, and inhabiting, at present, all the great divisions of the earth. An account, similar to our author's, of the name given to it by the American savages, is found in Kalm's Travels. "Mr. Bartram had found this plant in many places on his travels; but he did not know whether it was an original American plant, or whether the Europeans had brought it over. This doubt had its rise from the savages (who always had an extensive knowledge of the plants of the country) pretending that this plant never grew here before the arrival of the Europeans. They therefore gave it a name which signifies the Englishman's foot; for they say, that, where a European had walked, there this plant grew in his footsteps." — *Kalm's Travels into North America,* by Forster, vol. i. p. 92. But Dr. Pickering considers it possible, that, in North-west America at least, the plantain was introduced by the aborigines (Races of Man, pp. 317, 320): and, uncertain as this is admitted to be, the old vulgar names of

Black Henbane.[1]
Wormwood.[2]
Sharp pointed Dock.[3]
Patience.[4]

---

the plant in Northern languages — as *Wegerich* and *Wegetritt* of the German, *Weegblad* and *Weegbree* of the Dutch, *Veibred* of the Danish, and *Weybred* of old English, all pointing to the plantain's growing on ways trodden by man — suggest, perhaps, a far older supposed relation between this plant and the human foot than that mentioned above; and thus favor the derivation of the original Latin name (as old as Pliny, H. N., vol. xxv. 8, in § 39) from *planta*, the sole of the foot, — whether because the plantain is always trodden on, or, taking the termination *go* in *plantago*, as some philologists take it, to signify likeness (as doubtless in *lappago, mollugo, asperugo;* but this signification does not appear so clear in some other words with the like ending), because its leaves resemble the sole of the foot in flatness, breadth, marking, and so on. The possible derivation from planta, a plant, "*per excellentiam, quasi plantam præstantissimam*" (Tournef., Inst., vol. i. p. 128), though less open to question than that of Linnæus ("*planta tangenda,*" Phil. Bot., § 234), is certainly less significant than the other; which, with the statements (independent, so far as appears, of each other) of Josselyn and Kalm, if these may be relied on, seems to point to a very ancient co-incidence of thought, not unworthy of attention. Something else of the same sort is to be found in R. Williams, where he says (Key, *l. c.*, p. 218) that the Massachusetts Indians called the constellation of the Great Bear *mosk*, or *pawkunnawaw;* that is, the bear.

[1] Gerard, p. 353, — *Hyoscyamus niger*, L. *Adventive* only: having "escaped from gardens to roadsides," according to Dr. Gray (Man., p. 340); but "common amongst rubbish and by roadsides," in 1785 (Cutler, *l. c.*), and perhaps long known on the coasts of Massachusetts Bay.

[2] Broad-leaved wormwood, "our common and best-knowne wormwood" (Gerard, p. 1096), — *Artemisia absynthium*. L. "Roadsides and amongst rubbish," 1785, — *Cutler, l. c.* Omitted by Bigelow, and not very frequent.

[3] Gerard, p. 388. If this is to be taken for *Rumex acutus*, Sm. (Fl. Brit.), which seems not to be certain, it is now referable to *R. conglomeratus*, Murr., which is "sparingly introduced" with us, according to Gray (Man., p. 377). But it is more likely that Josselyn had *R. crispus*, L. (curled dock), in view: which is, I suppose, the "varietie" of sharp-pointed dock, "with crisped or curled leaves," of Johnson's Gerard, p. 387; and is the only mention of the species by those authors.

[4] Gerard, p. 389, — *Rumex Patientia*, L. This and the next were garden pot-

Bloodwort.[1]
And I fufpect *Adders Tongue.*[2]
Knot Grafs.[3]
Check weed.[4]
Compherie, with the white Flower.[5]
May weed, excellent for the Mother; fome of our *Englifh* Houfwives call it *Iron Wort,* and make a good Unguent for old Sores.[6]

---

herbs of repute: and, at p. 90, our author brings them in again as such; telling us that bloodwort grows "but sorrily," but patience "very pleasantly." This may very likely have crept out of some garden: but the great water-dock (*R. Hydrolapathum,* Huds.) is, says Gerard, "not unlike to the garden patience" (p. 390); and Dr. Gray says the same of the American variety of the former. — *Man.,* p. 377.

[1] Gerard, p. 390, — *Rumex sanguineus,* L., "sown for a pot-herb in most gardens" (Gerard); and so our author, p. 90. Linnæus took it to be originally American: but it is common in Europe; and Dr. Gray marks the American plant as naturalized. Dr. Torrey indicated the species as occurring about New York in 1819 (Catal. Pl., N.Y.); but New-England botanists do not appear to have recognized it. Josselyn's plant was perhaps the offcast of some garden.

[2] Gerard, p. 404. — Compare p. 42 of this; where our author more correctly reckons it among plants truly common to Europe and America.

[3] "Common knot-grasse" (Gerard. p. 565), — *Polygonum aviculare,* L. Common to all the great divisions of the earth, and reckoned indigenous in America. — *De Cand. Geogr. Bot.,* vol. i. p. 577; *Gray, Man.,* p. 373.

[4] There are many chickweeds in Gerard; but that most likely to have been in the author's view here is the universally known common chickweed, — the middle or small chickweed of Gerard, p. 611. This was "common in gardens and rich cultivated ground" in 1785. — *Cutler, l. c.* Few plants have spread so widely over the earth as *Stellaria media.*

[5] Great comfrey (Gerard, p. 806), — *Symphytum officinale,* L.: also in the list of garden herbs at p. 90. "Sometimes found growing wild," — *Cutler* (1785), *l. c.* Not admitted by Dr. Bigelow (Fl. Bost.), but included by Dr. Gray as an *adventive.* — *Man.,* p. 320.

[6] Gerard, p. 757. — *Maruta cotula* (L.), DC.; a naturalized member of our Flora, now become a very common ornament of roadsides; where Cutler notices it, also, in 1785.

The great *Clot Bur.*[1]
Mullin, with the white Flower.[2]

Q. What became of the influence of thofe Planets that produce and govern thefe Plants before this time!

I have now done with fuch Plants as grow wild in the Country in great plenty, (although I have not mentioned all) I fhall now in the Fifth place give you to under [87] ftand what *Englifh* Herbs we have growing in our Gardens that profper there as well as in their proper Soil, and of fuch as do not, and alfo of fuch as will not grow there at all.

---

5. *Of fuch Garden Herbs (amongſt us) as do thrive there, and of fuch as do not.*[3]

C*Abbidge* growes there exceeding well.
  Lettice.

---

[1] "Great burre-docke, or clott-burre" (Gerard, p. 809),—*Lappa major,* Gaertn. "About barns."— *Cutler* (1785), *l. c.*

[2] "White-floured mullein" (Gerard, p. 773),— perhaps *Verbascum Lychnitis,* L.; which is *adventive* in some parts of the United States (Gray, Man., p. 283), but is not otherwise known to have made its appearance in New England. Great mullein (*V. Thapsus,* L.) was "common" in Cutler's time. The moth-mullein (*V. Blattaria,* L.) he only knew "by roadsides in Lynn" (*l. c.,* p. 419). Other plants referable to this list of naturalized weeds are "wild sorrel," p. 42; *Polygonum Persicaria,* p. 43; St. John's wort, speedwell, chickweed, male fluellin, and clot-bur, p. 44; yarrow, and oak of Jerusalem, p. 46; pimpernel, and toadflax, p. 48; and wild purslain, and woad-waxen, p. 51. See also spearmint, and ground-ivy, p. 89; and elecampane, celandine, and tansy, p. 90.

[3] The earliest, almost the only account that we have of the gardens of our fathers, after they had settled themselves in their *New* England, and had tamed

Sorrel.
Parsley.
Marygold.

---

its rugged coasts to obedience to English husbandry. What with their garden beans, and Indian beans, and pease ("as good as ever I eat in England," says Higginson in 1629); their beets, parsnips, turnips, and carrots ("our turnips, parsnips, and carrots are both bigger and sweeter than is ordinary to be found in England," says the same reverend writer); their cabbages and asparagus,— both thriving, we are told, exceedingly; their radishes and lettuce; their sorrel, parsley, chervil, and marigold, for pot-herbs; and their sage, thyme, savory of both kinds, clary, anise, fennel, coriander, spearmint, and pennyroyal, for sweet herbs, — not to mention the Indian pompions and melons and squanter-squashes, "and other odde fruits of the country," — the first-named of which had got to be so well approved among the settlers, when Josselyn wrote in 1672, that what he calls "the ancient New-England standing dish" (we may well call it so now!) was made of them; and, finally, their pleasant, familiar flowers, lavender-cotton and hollyhocks and satin ("we call this herbe, in Norfolke, sattin," says Gerard; "and, among our women, it is called honestie") and gillyflowers, which meant pinks as well, and dear English roses, and eglantine, — yes, possibly, hedges of eglantine (p. 90 note), — surely the gardens of New England, fifty years after the settlement of the country, were as well stocked as they were a hundred and fifty years after. Nor were the first planters long behindhand in fruit. Even at his first visit, in 1639, our author was treated with "half a score very fair pippins," from the Governor's Island in Boston Harbor; though there was then, he says (Voyages, p. 29), "not one apple tree nor pear planted yet in no part of the countrey but upon that island." But he has a much better account to give in 1671: "The quinces, cherries, damsons, set the dames a work. Marmalad and preserved damsons is to be met with in every house. Our fruit-trees prosper abundantly,— apple-trees, pear-trees, quince-trees, cherry-trees, plum-trees, barberry-trees. I have observed, with admiration, that the kernels sown, or the succors planted, produce as fair and good fruit, without graffing, as the tree from whence they were taken. The countrey is replenished with fair and large orchards. It was affirmed by one Mr. Woolcut (a magistrate in Connecticut Colony), at the Captain's messe (of which I was), aboard the ship I came home in, that he made five hundred hogsheads of syder out of his own orchard in one year." — *Voyages*, p. 189-90. Our barberry-bushes, now so familiar inhabitants of the hedgerows of Eastern New England, should seem from this to have come, with the eglantines, from the gardens of the first settlers. Barberries "are planted in most of our English gardens," says Gerard.

French Mallowes.
Chervel.
Burnet.
Winter Savory.
Summer Savory.
Time.
Sage.
Carrats.
Parſnips of a prodigious ſize.
Red Beetes.
(88) *Radiſhes.*
Turnips.
Purſlain.[1]
Wheat.[2]
Rye.
Barley, which commonly degenerates into *Oats.*
Oats.

Peaſe of all ſorts, and the beſt in the World; I never heard of, nor did ſee in eight Years time, one Worm eaten Pea.
Garden Beans.[3]

---

[1] *Portulaca oleracea*,; L. β. *sativa*, L. (garden purslain). The wild variety is also reckoned by our author, in his list of plants, common to us and the Old World (p. 51).

[2] See Josselyn's Voyages, p. 188.

[3] *Vicia Faba*, Willd., of which the Windsor bean is a variety. The author compares it, at p. 56, with kidney-beans (*Phaseolus vulgaris*, L.), called Indian beans by the first settlers, who had them from the savages, to the advantage of the last-mentioned sort; which probably soon drove the other out of our gardens. — Compare Cobbett's American Gardener, p. 105.

Naked Oats,[1] there called *Silpee,* an excellent grain ufed infteed of Oat Meal, they dry it in an Oven, or in a Pan upon the fire, then beat it fmall in a Morter.

Another ftanding Dijh in New-England.

And when the Milk is ready to boil, they put into a pottle of Milk about ten or twelve fpoonfuls of this Meal, fo boil it leafurely, ftirring of it every foot, leaft it burn too; when it is almoft boiled enough, they hang the Kettle up higher, and let it ftew only, in fhort time it will thicken like a Cuftard; they feafon it [89] with a little Sugar and Spice, and fo ferve it to the Table in deep Bafons, and it is altogether as good as a White-pot.

For People weakned with long Sicknefs.

It exceedingly nourifheth and ftrengthens people weakned with long Sicknefs.

Sometimes they make Water Gruel with it, and fome-

---

[1] Gerard, p. 75, — *Avena nuda,* L.; derived from common oats (*A. sativa,* L.) according to Link; and also (in Gerard's time, and even later) in cultivation. It was called pillcorn, or peelcorn, because the grains, when ripe, drop naked from the husks. But is it not possible that our author's *Silpee* (comparable with *apee,* a leaf; *toopee,* a root; *uhpee,* a bow, in the Micmac language, — *Mass. Hist. Coll.,* vol. vi., pp. 20, 24) was really the American name of the well-known water-oats, or Canada rice, — *Zizania aquatica,* L.; the deciduous grains of which are said to afford "a very good meal" (Loudon, Encycl., p. 788), with the qualities of rice? — See *Bigel., Fl. Bost.,* edit. 3, p. 369. This has long been used by our savages; but I have not met with any mention of it in the early writers. The "standing dish in New England" has its interest, if it were really made of Canada rice.

times thicken their Flefh Broth either with this or *Hom-miney*, if it be for Servants.

Spear Mint.[1]
Rew, will hardly grow.
Fetherfew profpereth exceedingly.
Southern Wood, is no Plant for this Country. Nor,
Rofemary. Nor
Bayes.[2]
White Satten groweth pretty well, fo doth
Lavender Cotton.[3] But
Lavender is not for the climate.
Penny Royal.
Smalledge.
Ground Ivy, or *Ale Hoof.*[4]
Gilly Flowers will continue two Years.[5]

[90] *Fennel* muft be taken up, and kept in a warm Cellar all Winter.

---

[1] Gerard, p. 680, — *Mentha viridis*, L. It perhaps soon became naturalized. "In moist ground" (1785). — *Cutler, l. c.*

[2] Perhaps only an inference of the author's, from the southern origin of these three shrubs. Lavender also belongs naturally to a warmer climate.

[3] Gerard, p. 1109, — *Santolina Chamæ Cyparissus*, L.

[4] Gerard, p. 856. — *Glechoma hederacea*, L.; once of great medicinal repute: which accounts for our author's finding it, as it should seem, among garden-herbs. It has become naturalized and very familiar in New England. Cutler finds it wild in 1785. Mr. Bentham refers it to *Nepeta*, but substitutes a new specific name for that given by Linnæus, which is based on the ancient names, and has at least the right of priority.

[5] "Gilliflowers thrive exceedingly there, and are very large. The collibuy, or humming-bird, is much pleased with them." — *Josselyn's Voyages*, p. 188.

S

Houfleck profpereth notably.

Holly hocks.

Enula Campana, in two Years time the Roots rot.[1]

Comferie, with white Flowers.

Coriander,   and

Dill.   and

Annis thrive exceedingly, but *Annis Seed*, as alfo the Seed of *Fennel* feldom come to maturity; the Seed of *Annis* is commonly eaten with a fly.

Clary never lafts but one Summer, the Roots rot with the Froft.

Sparagus thrives exceedingly, fo does

Garden Sorrel, and

Sweet Bryer, or *Eglantine.*[2]

Bloodwort but forrily, but

Patience,[3] and

Englifh Rofes, very pleafantly.[4]

---

[1] Elecampane (Gerard, p. 793), — *Inula Helenium*, L. "Roadsides" (1785), — *Cutler, l. c.;* and now extensively naturalized in New England.

[2] Gerard, p. 1272, — *Rosa rubiginosa*, L.; and *R. micrantha*, Sm. Since naturalized, especially in Eastern New England, and not uncommon on roadsides and in pastures. First indicated as a member of our Flora by Bigelow in 1824. — *Fl. Bost., in loc.* "Eglantine, or sweet-bryer, is best sowen with juniperberries, — two or three to one eglantine-berry, put into a hole made with a stick. The next year, separate and remove them to your banks. In three years' time, they will make a hedge as high as a man; which you may keep thick and handsome with cutting." — *Josselyn's Voyages*, p. 188. And what next goes before seems to show that the author picked up this information here; which is not uninteresting.

[3] See p. 86.

[4] Brier-rose, or hep-tree (Gerard, p. 1270); "also called *Rosa canina*, which is a plant so common and well knowne, that it were to small purpose to use many

Celandine, by the West Country men called *Kenning Wort*, grows but flowly.[1]

Mufchata, as well as in *England*.

Dittander, or *Pepper Wort*, flourifheth notably, and fo doth.

Tanfie.[2]

Mufk Mellons are better than our *Englifh*, and.

[91] *Cucumbers*.

Pompions, there be of feveral kinds, fome proper to the Country,[3] they are dryer then our *Englifh* Pompions, and better tafted; you may eat them green.

---

words in the description thereof: for even children with great delight eat the berries thereof, when they be ripe, — make chaines and other prettie gewgawes of the fruit; cookes and gentlewomen make tarts, and such like dishes, for pleasure thereof," &c. (Gerard, *l. c.*). *Rosa canina*, L., was once the collective name of what are now understood as many distinct species; but that which still retains the name of dog-rose is reckoned the finest of native English roses. This familiar plant may well have been reared with tender interest in some New-England gardens of Josselyn's day; but it did not make a new home here, like the eglantine. Cutler gives the name of dog-rose to the Carolina rose, — *R. Carolina*, L., — which it has not kept; and he also makes it equivalent to the officinal *R. canina*. Our Flora will possibly one day include one or two other garden-roses. A damask rose is well established and spreading rapidly in mowing-land of the writer's, and elsewhere on roadsides of this country; and that general favorite, the cinnamon-rose, which is now naturalized in England, may yet become wild with us.

[1] Great celandine (Gerard, p. 1069), as the west-country name of kenningwort — that is, sight-wort — makes manifest; the juice being once thought to be " good to sharpen the sight," — *Chelidonium majus*, L. Small celandine (*Ranunculus Ficaria*, L.) was quite another thing. The former had got to be " common by fences and amongst rubbish " in 1785 (Cutler, *l. c.*), and is now naturalized in Eastern New England.

[2] Gerard, p. 650, — *Tanacetum vulgare*, L. In "pastures" (1785). — *Cutler, l. c.* Now widely naturalized in New England.

[3]*See p. 57, note. " The ancient New-England standing dish " was doubtless far better than Gerard's fried pompions (p. 921), and has more than held its own.

The ancient New-England ſtanding Diſh.

But the Houſwives manner is to ſlice them when ripe,
and cut them into dice, and ſo fill a pot with them of two
or three Gallons, and ſtew them upon a gentle fire a whole
day, and as they ſink, they fill again with freſh Pompions,
not putting any liquor to them; and when it is ſtew'd
enough, it will look like bak'd Apples; this they Diſh,
putting Butter to it, and a little Vinegar, (with ſome Spice,
as Ginger, &c.) which makes it tart like an Apple, and ſo
ſerve it up to be eaten with Fiſh or Fleſh: It provokes
Urin extreamly and is very windy.

---

[92] Sixthly and laſtly,

Of Stones, Minerals, Metals and Earths.[1]

A S firſt, the *Emrald* which grows in flat Rocks, and is
very good.

Rubies, which here are very watry.

---

[1] "For such commodities as lie under ground, I cannot, out of mine own
experience or knowledge, say much; having taken no great notice of such things;
but it is certainly reported that there is iron-stone; and the Indians informed us
that they can lead us to the mountains of black-lead; and have shown us lead-
ore, if our small judgment in such things does not deceive us; and though nobody
dare confidently conclude, yet dare they not utterly deny, but that the Spaniard's-
bliss may lie hid in the barren mountains. Such as have coasted the country
affirm that they know where to fetch sea-coal, if wood were scarce. There is
plenty of stone, both rough and smooth, useful for many things; with quarries of
slate, out of which they get coverings for houses; with good clay, whereof they

I have heard a ſtory of an *Indian*, that found a ſtone, up in the Country, by a great Pond as big as an Egg, that in a dark Night would give a light to read by; but I take it to be but a ſtory.

Diamond, which are very brittle, and therefore of little worth.

Cryſtal, called by our Weſt Country Men the *Kenning Stone*; by *Sebegug* Pond is found in conſiderable quantity, not far from thence is a Rock of Cryſtal called the *Mooſe* Rock, becauſe in ſhape like a *Mooſe*,   and

Muſcovy Glaſs, both white and purple of reaſonable content.

---

make tiles and bricks and pavements for their necessary uses. For the country it is well watered as any land under the sun; every family, or every two families, having a spring of sweet water betwixt them; which is far different from the waters of England, being not so sharp, but of a fatter substance, and of a more jetty colour. . . . Those that drink it be as healthful, fresh, and lusty as they that drink beer." — *Wood, New-Eng. Prospect,* chap. v. "The humour and justness of" this writer's "account recommend him," says the editor of 1764, "to every candid mind." There is certainly no view of New England, as it was at its settlement, that surpasses Wood's in understanding, and homeborn English truth, not always without beauty. What he says in this place of " quarries of slate" points to a very early discovery. Higginson says, in 1629 (New-Eng. Plantation, *l. c.,* p. 118), " Here is plenty of slates at the Isle of Slate in Masathulets Bay:" and there is a court order of July 2, 1633, granting "to Tho: Lambe, of slate in Slate Ileand, 10 poole towards the water-side, and 5 poole into the land, for three yeares: payeing the yearely rent of ijs. vjd." — *Mass. Col. Rec.,* vol. i. p. 106. There are other later grants of the same island, which "lies between Bumkin Island and Weymouth River." — *Pemberton, Desc. Bost., Mass. Hist. Coll.,* vol. iii. p. 297. Josselyn, in his Voyages, p. 46, says that tables of slate could be got out (he does not tell us where), " long enough for a dozen men to sit at." Argillaceous slate is, according to Dr. Hitchcock, " the predominating rock on the outermost of these islands; " and he adds, that " there can be but little doubt that the peninsula of Boston has a foundation" of this rock. — *Report on Geol. of Mass.,* p. 270.

Black Lead.[1]
Bole Armoniack.
[93] Red and Yellow *Oker*.
Terra Sigilla.
Vitriol.
Antimony.
Arfnick, too much.
Lead.[2]
Tin.
Tin Glafs.
Silver.

Iron, in abundance, and as good bog Iron as any in the World.

Copper. It is reported that the French have a *Copper* Mine at *Port Royal*, that yieldeth them twelve Ounces of pure *Copper* out of a Pound of *Oar*.

---

[1] "Mr. John Winthrope, jun., is granted yᵉ hill at Tantousq, about 60 miles westward, in which the black-leade is; and liberty to purchase some land there of the Indians" (13th November, 1644). — *Mass. Col. Rec.*, vol. ii. p. 82; and *Savage, in Winthrop, N. E.*, vol. ii. p. 213, note. The place mentioned is what is now Sturbridge; which is called "the most important locality" of black-lead in Massachusetts, by Dr. Hitchcock. — *Geol.*, pp. 47, 395.

[2] "The mountains and rocky hills are richly furnished with mines of lead, silver, copper, tin, and divers sorts of minerals, branching out even to their summits; where, in small crannies, you may meet with threds of perfe*ct* silver: yet have the English no maw to open any of them;" and so forth. — *Josselyn's Voyages*, p. 44.

I fhall conclude this Section with a ftrange Cure effected upon a Drummers Wife, much afflicted with a Wolf in her Breaft; the poor Woman lived with her Husband at a Town called by the *Indians*, *Cafco*; but by the *Englifh*, *Famouth*; where for fome time fhe fwaged the Pain of her Sore, by bathing it with ftrong Malt Beer, which it would [94] fuck in greedily, as if fome living Creature : When fhe could come by no more Beer, (for it was brought from *Bofton*, along the Coafts by Merchants,) fhe made ufe of *Rhum*, a ftrong Water drawn from Sugar Canes, with which it was lull'd a fleep; at laft, (to be rid of it altogether) fhe put a quantity of *Arfnick* to the *Rhum*, and bathing of it as formerly, fhe utterly deftroyed it, and Cured her felf; but her kind Husband, who fucked out the Poyfon as the Sore was healing, loft all his Teeth, but without further danger or inconvenience.

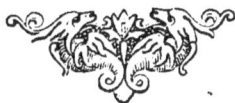

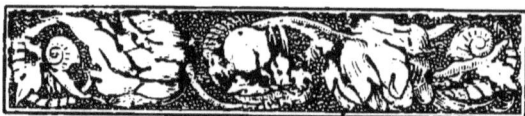

[95] *An* ADDITION *of* ſome *RARITIES overſlipt.*

THe *Star Fiſh,*[1] having fine points like a- Star, the whole Fiſh no bigger than the Palm of a Mans hand, of a tough ſubſtance like leather, and about an Inch in thickneſs, whitiſh underneath, and of the Colour of a Cucumber above, and ſomewhat ruff: When it is warm in ones hand, you may perceive a ſtiff motion, turning down one point, and thruſting up another: It is taken to be poyſonous; they are very common, and found thrown up on the Rocks by the Sea ſide.

Sea Bream, which are plentifully taken upon the Sea Coaſts, their Eyes are accounted rare Meat, whereupon the proverbial compariſon, *It is worth a Sea Breams Eye.*[2]

---

[1] *Asterias rubens,* L. — *Gould, Report on Invert.,* p. 345.
[2] See the chapter on Fiſhes, p. 23, for this and the others here spoken of.

[96] *Blew Fish*, or *Horse*, I did never fee any of them in *England*; they are as big ufually as the *Salmon*, and better Meat by far: It is common in *New-England* and efteemed the beft fort of Fifh next to *Rock Cod*.

Cat Fish, having a round Head, and great glaring Eyes like a Cat: They lye for the moft part in holes of Rocks, and are difcovered by their Eyes: It is an excelling Fifh.

Munk Fish, a flat Fifh like fcate, having a hood like a Fryers Cowl.

Clam, or *Clamp*, a kind of *Shell Fish*, a white Mufcle.

An Acharifton, For Pin and Web.

Sheath Fish, which are there very plentiful, a delicate Fifh, as good as a *Prawn*, covered with a thin Shell like the fheath of a Knife, and of the colour of a *Mufcle*.

Which fhell Calcin'd and Pulveriz'd, is excellent to take off a Pin and Web, or [97] any kind of Filme growing over the Eye.

Morfe, or *Sea Horfe*, having a great Head, wide Jaws, armed with Tufhes as white as Ivory, of body as big as a Cow, proportioned like a Hog, of brownifh bay, fmooth skin'd and impenetrable; they are frequent at the Ifle of

T

Sables, their Teeth are worth eight Groats the Pound; the beſt Ivory being Sold but for half the Money.[1]

For Poyſon.
It is very good againſt Poyſon.

For the Cramp.
As alſo for the Cramp, made into Rings.

For the Piles.
And a ſecret for the *Piles,* if a wiſe Man have the order-ing of it.

The *Manaty,* a Fiſh as big as a Wine pipe, moſt excel-lent Meat; bred in the Rivers of *Hiſpaniola* in the *Weſt Indies*; it hath Teats, and nouriſheth its young ones with Milk; it is of a green Colour, and taſteth like Veal.

[98] For the Stone Collick.
There is a Stone taken out of the Head that is rare for the *Stone* and *Collect.*

---

[1] "Numerous about the Isle of Sables; i.e., the Sandy Isle." — *Voyages.* p. 106. "Mr. Graves" (year 1635) "in the 'James,' and Mr. Hodges in the 'Re-becka,' set sail for the Isle of Sable for sea-horse, which are there in great num-ber," &c. — *Winthrop's N. E., by Savage,* vol. i. p. 162. And I cite one other mention of this pursuit: "Eastward is the Isle of Sables; whither one John Webb, *alias* Evered (an active man), with his company, are gone, with commis-sion from the Bay to get sea-horse teeth and oyle." — *Lechford's Newes from New England* (1642), *Mass. Hist. Coll.,* vol. iii. 3d series, p. 100. The Magda-len Islands, in the Gulf of St. Lawrence, are the most southern habitat of the animal spoken of by Godman. — *Amer. Nat. Hist.,* vol. i. p. 249.

To provoke Urine.

Their Bones beat to a Powder and drank with convenient Liquors, is a gallant Urin provoking Medicine.

For Wound and Bruise.

An *Indian*, whose Knee was bruised with a fall, and the
Skin and Flesh strip'd down to the middle of the Calf of
his Leg; Cured himself with *Water Lilly* Roots boyled
and stamped.[1]

For Swellings of the Foot.

An *Indian* Webb, her Foot being very much swell'd
and inflamed, asswaged the swelling, and took away the
inflamation with our Garden or *English Patience*, the Roots
roasted. *f. Cataplas. Anno* 1670. *June* 28.

To dissolve a Scirrhous Tumour.

An *Indian* dissolv'd a *Scirrhous Tumour* in the Arm and
Hip, with a fomentation of Tobacco, applying afterwards
the Herb stamp'd betwixt two stones.

---

[1] Compare Cutler (Account of Indig. Veg., *l. c.*, p. 456) and Wood and Bache
(Dispens., p. 1369).

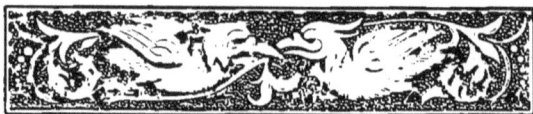

A

DESCRIPTION

OF AN

INDIAN SQUA.[1]

NOw (gentle Reader) having trefpaffed upon your patience a long while in the perufing of thefe rude Obfervations, I fhall, to make you amends, prefent you by way of Divertifement, or Recreation, with a Coppy of Verfes made fometime fince upon the Picture of a young

---

[1] The author has something to the same effect in his Voyages, p. 124; but Wood's account of the Indian women (New-England's Prospect, part ii. chap. xx.) is far better worth reading. Both appreciated, in one way or another, their savage neighbors. Wood has a pleasant touch at the last. "These women," he says, "resort often to the English houses, where *pares cum paribus congregatæ,* — in sex, I mean, — they do somewhat ease their misery by complaining, and seldom part without a relief. If her husband come to seek for his squaw, and begin to bluster, the English woman betakes her to her arms, which are the warlike ladle and the scalding liquors, threatning blistering to the naked runaway, who is soon expelled by such liquid comminations. In a word, to conclude this woman's history, their love to the English hath deserved no small esteem; ever presenting them something that is either rare or desired, — as strawberries, hurtleberries, rasberries, gooseberries, cherries, plumbs, fish, and other such gifts as their poor treasury yields them " (*l. c.*). And, if Lechford's Newes from New England (*l. supra c.*, p. 103) can be trusted, the savages became "much the . kinder to their wives by the example of the English."

and handfome *Gypfie*, not improperly transferred upon the *Indian SQUA*, or Female *Indian*, trick'd up in all her bravery.

The Men are fomewhat Horfe Fac'd, and generally Faucious, *i. e.* without Beards; but the Women many of them [100] have very good Features; feldome without a *Come to me*, or *Cos Amoris*, in their Countenance; all of them black Eyed, having even fhort Teeth, and very white; their Hair black, thick and long, broad Breafted; hand-fome ftreight Bodies, and flender, confidering their con-ftant loofe habit: Their limbs cleanly, ftraight, and of a convenient ftature, generally, as plump as Partridges, and faving here and there one, of a modeft deportment.

Their Garments are a pair of Sleeves of Deer, or Moofe skin dreft, and drawn with lines of feveral Colours into Afiatick Works, with Buskins of the fame, a fhort Mantle of Trading Cloath, either Blew or Red, faftened with a knot under the Chin, and girt about the middle with a Zone, wrought with white and blew Beads into pretty Works; of thefe Beads they have Bracelets for their Neck and Arms, and Links to hang in their Ears, and a fair Table curioufly made up with Beads likewife, to wear before their Breaft; their Hair they Combe backward, and tye it up fhort with a Border, about two handfulls broad, [101] wrought in Works as the other with their Beads: But enough of this.

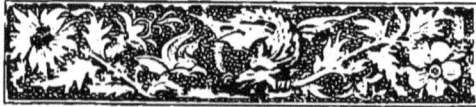

The *P O E M.*

WHether *White or Black be beſt*
    Call your Senſes to the queſt;
    And your touch ſhall quickly tell
    The Black in ſoftneſs doth excel,
And in ſmoothneſs; but the Ear,
What, can that a Colour hear?
No, but 'tis your Black ones Wit
That doth catch, and captive it.
And if Slut and Fair be one,
Sweet and Fair, there can be none:
Nor can ought ſo pleaſe the taſt
As what's brown and lovely dreſt:
And who'll ſay, that that is beſt
To pleaſe ones Senſe, diſpleaſe the reſt?
[102] Maugre then all that can be ſed
In flattery of White and Red:
Thoſe flatterers themſelves muſt ſay
That darkneſs was before the Day:
And ſuch perfection here appears
It neither Wind nor Sun-ſhine fears.

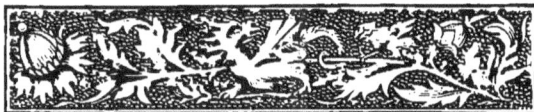

A

[103] Chronological TABLE

Of the most remarkable passages in that part of 'America, *known to us by the name of* NEW-ENGLAND.*[1]

A *Nno Dom.* 1492. *Chriſt. Columbus* diſcovered *America.*

1516. The Voyage of Sir *Thomas Pert,* Vice Admiral of *England,* and Sir *Sebaſtian Cabota* to *Brazile, &c.*

1527. *New-found-Land,* diſcovered by the *Engliſh.*

1577. Sir *Francis Drake* began his Voyage about the *World.*

---

[1] In the author's Voyages, this chronological table is greatly extended; beginning with "*Anno Mundi,* 3720," and ending with A.D. 1674.

Anno Dom.

[104] 1585. *Nova Albion* difcovered by Sir *Francis Drake*, and by him fo Named.

1585. *April* 9. Sir *Richard Greenevile* was fent by Sir *Walter Rawleigh* with a Fleet of Seven Sail to *Virginia*, and was ftiled the General of *Virginia*.

1586. Captain *Thomas Candifh*, a *Suffolk* Gentleman, began his Voyage round about the World, with three Ships paft the Streights of *Magellan*, burn'd and ranfack'd in the entry of *Chile, Peru*, and *New-Spain*, near the great Ifland *Callifornia* in the South Sea; and returned to *Plymouth* with a precious Booty *Anno Dom.* 1588. *September* the 8*th*; being the third fince *Magellan* that circuited the Earth.

1588. Sir *Walter Rawleigh* firft difcovered *Virginia*, by him fo Named, in honour of our Virgin Queen.

1595. Sir *Walter Rawleigh* difcovered *Guiana:*

[105] 1606. A Collony fent to *Virginia*.

1614. *Bermudas* Planted.

1618. The blazing Star; then *Plymouth* Plantation began in *New-England*.[1]

---

[1] Set right by the author in Voyages, p. 248.

Anno Dom.

1628. The *Maffachufets* Colony Planted, and *Salem* the firft Town therein Built.[1]

1629. The firft Church gathered in this Colony was at *Salem*; from which Year to this prefent Year, is 43 Years.

In the compafs of thefe Years, in this Colony, there hath been gathered Fourty Churches, and 120 Towns built in all the Colonies of *New-England*.

---

[1] The author, in the "chronological obfervations" appended to his Voyages, enlarges this, but confounds Conant's Plantation at Cape Ann, and Endicott's, as follows: "1628. Mr. John Endicot arrived in New England with some number of people, and set down first by Cape Ann, at a place called afterwards Glofter; but their abiding-place was at Salem, where they built the first town in the Maffachufets Patent. . . . 1629. Three ships arrived at Salem, bringing a great number of paffengers from England. . . . Mr. Endicot chofen Governour." The next year, Joffelyn continues as follows: "1630. The 10th of July, John Winthrop, Efq., and the Affiftants, arrived in New England with the patent for the Maffachufetts. . . . John Winthrop, Efq., chofen Governour for the remainder of the year; Mr. Thomas Dudley, Deputy-Governour; Mr. Simon Broadftreet, Secretary." — *Voyages*, p. 252. The title of Governor was used anciently, as it ftill is elfewhere, in a looser sense than has been ufual in New England; and derived all the dignity that it had from the character and confiderableness of the government. Conant and Endicott were directors or governors of settlements in the Maffachusetts Bay before Winthrop's arrival; but when the Maffachusetts Company in London proceeded. on the 20th October, 1629, to carry into effect their refolution to transfer their government to this country, — and chose accordingly Winthrop to be their Governor; Humphrey, their Deputy-Governor; and Endicot and others. Affiftants (Young. Chron. of Mass., p. 102), — the record appears sufficient evidence that they had in view something quite different from the fifhing plantation which Conant had had charge of at Cape Ann, or the little fociety ("in all, not much above fifty or fixty perfons," fays White's Relation in Young. Chron., p. 13: which the editor. from Higginfon's narrative, raifes to "about a hundred") "of which Mafter Endecott was sent out Governour" (White, *l. c.*) at Naumkeak.

U

Anno Dom.

The Church of Chrift at *Plymouth*, was Planted in *New-England* Eight Years before others.

1630.   The Governour and Affiftants [106] arrived with their Pattent for the *Maffachufets*.

1630.   The Lady *Arabella* in *New-England.*

1630.   When the Government was eftablifhed, they Planted on *Noddles* Ifland.[1]

1631.   Captain *John Smith* Governour of *Virginia*, and Admiral of *New-England*, Dyed.

1631.   Mr. *Mavericke* Minifter at *Dorchefter* in *New-England.*[2]

1631.   *John Winthorpe* Efq; chofen the firft time Governour, he was eleven times Governour; fome fay Nineteen times; eleven Years together; the other Years by intermiffion.

1631.   *John Wilfon* Paftor of *Charles* Town.[2]

[107] 1631.   Sir *R. Saltingftall* at *Water Town* came into *New-England.*[2]

---

[1] That is, Noddle's Ifland was already planted on (by Mr. Maverick) when the government was eftablifhed. — Compare Johnson, cited by Prince, N. E. Chronol., edit. 2, p. 30S, note.

[2] The date set right in Prince, N. E. Chronol., p. 367.

Anno Dom.

1631. Mr. *Rog. Harlackinden* was a Majeftrate, and a Leader of their Military Forces.[1]

Dr. *Wilfon* gave ·1000 *l.* to *New-England*, with which they ftored themfelves with great Guns.[2]

1633. Mr. *Thomas Hooker*, Mr. *Haynes*, and Mr. *John Cotton*, came over together in one Ship.

1634. The Country was really placed in a pofture of War, to be in readinefs at all times.

1635. *Hugh Peters* went over for *New-England*.

1636. *Connecticut* Colony Planted.

[108] 1637. The *Pequites* Wars, in which were Slain Five or Six Hundred *Indians*.

Minifters that have come from *England*, chiefly in the Ten firft Years, Ninety Four: Of which returned Twenty Seven: Dyed in the Country Thirty Six: Yet alive in the Country Thirty One.

---

[1] The date corrected in Prince, N. E. Chronol., edit. 2, p. 367.

[2] Compare Prince, p. 367, and Mass. Col. Rec., vol. i. p. 128. "The will," says Dr. Mather, "because it bequeathed a thousand pounds to New England, gave satisfaction unto our Mr. Wilson; though it was otherwise injurious to himself." — *Magnalia*, vol. iii. p. 45, *cit.* Davis, *in Morton's Memorial*, p. 334, note.

The Number of Ships that tranfported Paffengers to *New-England* in thefe times, was 298. fuppofed: Men, Women, and Children, as near as can be gheffed 21200.

1637. The firft Synod at *Cambridge* in *New-England*, where the *Antinomian* and *Famaliftical* Errors were confuted; 80 Errors now amongft the *Maffachufets*.

1638. *New-Haven* Colony began.

Mrs. *Hutchinfon* and her erronious companions banifhed the *Maffachufets* Colony.

[109] A terrible Earth quake throughout the Country.[1]
Mr. *John Harvard*, the Founder of *Harvard* College (at *Cambridge* in *New-England*) Deceafed, gave 700 *l.* to the erecting of it.

1639. Firft Printing at *Cambridge* in *New-England*.

1639. A very fharp Winter in *New-England*.

1642. *Harvard* College Founded with a publick Library.

Minifters bred in *New-England*, and (excepting about

---

[1] Compare Winthrop, N.E., vol. i. p. 265; Johnson's Wonder-working Prov. lib. ii. c. 12, *cit.* Savage; and Morton's Memorial, by Davis, p. 209, and note, p. 289.

Anno Dom.

10,) in *Harvard* College 132; of which dyed in the Country 10; now living 81; removed to *England* 41.

1643. The firſt combination of the Four United Colonies, *viz. Plymouth, Maſſachuſets, Connecticut,* and *New-Haven.*

[110] 1646. The ſecond Synod at *Cambridge,* touching the duty and power of Majeſtrates in matters of Religion: Secondly, the nature and power of Synods.

Mr. *Eliot* firſt Preached to the *Indians* in their Native Language.

1647. Mr. *Thomas Hooker* Died.

1648. The third Synod at *Cambridge,* publiſhing the Platform of Diſcipline.

1649. Mr. *John Winthorpe* Governour, now Died.

This Year a ſtrange multitude of *Caterpillers* in *New-England.* [1]

Thrice ſeven Years after the Planting of the *Engliſh* in *New-England,* the *Indians* of *Maſſachuſets* being 30000 able Men were brought to 300.

---

[1] Morton's Memorial, by Davis, p. 244.

1651. *Hugh Peters,* and Mr. *Wells* came for *England.*

[111] 1652. Mr. *John Cotton* Dyed.

1653. The great Fire in *Boston* in *New-England.*

Mr. *Thomas Dudley,* Governour of the *Massachusets,* Dyed this Year.

1654. *Major Gibbons* Died in *New-England.*

1655. *Jamaica* Taken by the *English.*

1657. The *Quakers* arrived in *New-England,* at *Plymouth.*

1659. Mr. *Henry Dunster* the first President of *Harvard* College now Dyed.

1661. Major *Atherton* Dyed in *New-England.*

1663. Mr. *John Norton* Pastor of *Boston* in *New-England,* Dyed suddenly.

[112] Mr. *Samuel Stone,* Teacher of *Hartford* Church, Dyed this Year.

1664. The whole *Bible* Printed in the *Indian* Language finished.

Anno Dom.

The *Manadaes*, called New *Amſterdam*, now called New *York*; furrendred up to His Majeſties Commiſſion-ers (for the fettling of the refpective Colonies in *New-England, viz.* Sir *Robert Carr*, Collonel *Nicols*, Collonel *Cartwright*, and Mr. *Samuel Mavericke*,) in *September*, after thirteen Dayes the Fort of *Arania*, now *Albania*; twelve Dayes after that, the Fort *Awſapha*; then *de la Ware* Caſtle Man'd with *Dutch* and *Sweeds*; the Three firſt Forts and Towns being Built upon the great River *Mohegan*, otherwife called *Hudſons* River.

In *September* appeared a great Comet for the ſpace of three Months.[1]

1665. Mr. *John Indicot*, Governour of the *Maſſachu-ſets* Dyed.

[113] A thoufand Foot fent this Year by the *French* King to *Canada*.

Captain *Davenport* killed with Lightning at the Caſtle by *Boſton* in *New-England*, and feveral Wounded.

---

[1] 1664, " December, a great and dreadful comet, or blazing star, appeared in the south-eaſt in New England for the space of three moneths; which was ac-companied with many sad effects, — great mildews blasting in the countrey the next summer." — *Joſſelyn's Voyages, Chronol. Obs.*, p. 273; and see p. 245 of the same for a fuller account. — Compare Morton's Memorial, by Davis, p. 304. As to the blaſting and mildew of 1665, see the same, p. 317; and that of 1664, p. 309.

1666. The *Small Pox* at *Boston.* Seven flain by Lightning, and divers Burnt: This Year also *New-England* had caft away, and taken 31 Veffels, and fome in 1667.

1667. Mr. *John Wilson* Paftor of *Boston* Dyed, aged 79 Years.

1670. At a place called *Kenibunck,* which is in the Province of *Meyne,* a Colony belonging to the Heir of that Honourable Knight Sir *Ferdinando Gorges;* not far from the River fide, a piece of Clay Ground was thrown up by a Mineral vapour (as we fuppofed) over the tops of high Oaks that grew between it and the River, into the River, ftopping the courfe thereof, and leaving a hole two Yards fquare, wherein were thoufands of [114] Clay Bullets as big as Mufquet Bullets, and pieces of Clay in fhape like the Barrel of a Mufquet.[1]

---

[1] See Josselyn's Voyages, p. 204 and p. 277, where the "hole" is said to have been, not "two," but "forty, yards square:" and we are farther told that "the like accident fell out at Casco, one and twenty miles from it to the eastward, much about the same time; and fish, in some ponds in the countrey, thrown up dead upon the banks. — supposed likewise to be kill'd with mineral vapours." Hubbard (Hist. N.E., chap. 75) tells this, partly in the same words with the account in the Voyages, and adds, "All the whole town of Wells are witnesses of the truth of this relation; and many others have seen sundry of these clay pellets, which the inhabitants have shown to their neighbours of other towns." And compare also the following, at p. 189 of the Voyages: "In 1669, the pond that lyeth between Watertown and Cambridge cast its fish dead upon the shore; forc't by a mineral vapour, as was conjectured."

Anno Dom.

1671.   Elder *Penn* dyed at *Boſton*.

1672.   Mr. *Richard Bellingham*, Governour of the *Maſſachuſets* in *New-England*.

.

NOTE.

The book is reprinted literally, except in the following items : —

Page 86. line 21, "Planets" is corrected to Plants.

Page 104, line 4, "Richards" is printed Richard; and, line 5, "Water" is corrected to Walter.

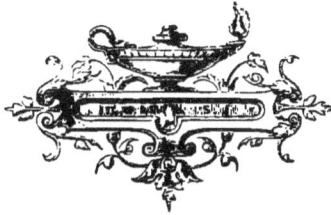

www.ingramcontent.com/pod-product-compliance
Lightning Source LLC
Chambersburg PA
CBHW020541270326
41927CB00006B/677